Older people and community care

RETHINKING AGEING SERIES

Series editor: Brian Gearing
                 School of Health and Social Welfare
                 The Open University

The rapid growth in ageing populations in Britain and other countries has led to a dramatic increase in academic and professional interest in the subject. Over the past decade this has led to the publication of many research studies which have stimulated new ideas and fresh approaches to understanding old age. At the same time, there has been concern about continued neglect of ageing and old age in the education and professional training of most workers in health and social services, and about inadequate dissemination of the new information and ideas about ageing to a wider public.

This series aims to fill a gap in the market for accessible, up-to-date studies of important issues in ageing. Each book will focus on a topic of current concern addressing two fundamental questions: what is known about this topic? And what are the policy, service and practice implications of our knowledge? Authors will be encouraged to develop their own ideas, drawing on case material, and their own research, professional or personal experience. The books will be interdisciplinary, and written in clear, non-technical language which will appeal to a broad range of students, academics and professionals with a common interest in ageing and age care.

Current and forthcoming titles:
Simon Biggs *et al.*: **Elder abuse in perspective**
Ken Blakemore and Margaret Boneham: **Age, race and ethnicity: A comparative approach**
Joanna Bornat (ed.): **Reminiscence reviewed: Perspectives, evaluations, achievements**
Joanna Bornat and Maureen Cooper: **Older learners**
Bill Bytheway: **Ageism**
Beverley Hughes: **Older people and community care: Critical theory and practice**
Anne Jamieson: **Comparing policies of care for older people**
Sheila Peace *et al.*: **Re-evaluating residential care**
Moyra Sidell: **Health in old age: Myth, mystery and management**
Andrew Sixsmith: **Quality of life: Rethinking well-being in old age**
Robert Slater: **The psychology of growing old: Looking forward**

Older people and community care
Critical theory and practice

BEVERLEY HUGHES

OPEN UNIVERSITY PRESS
Buckingham · Philadelphia

Open University Press
Celtic Court
22 Ballmoor
Buckingham
MK18 1XW

and
1900 Frost Road, Suite 101
Bristol, PA 19007, USA

First Published 1995

A catalogue record of this book is available from the British Library

ISBN 0 335 19157 6 (hb)   0 335 19156 8 (pb)

Library of Congress Cataloging-in-Publication Data

Hughes, Beverley, 1950–
        Older people and community care: critical theory and practice/[Beverly Hughes].
            p.   cm. – (Rethinking ageing series)
        Includes bibliographical references and index.
        ISBN 0–335–19157–6. (hb) ISBN 0–335–19156–8 (pb)
        1. Community health services for the aged – Great Britain.   2. Ageism.
I. Title.   II. Series.
RA564.8.H84   1995
362.1'9897'00941–dc20   95–14731
                                                                                                    CIP

Typeset by Type Study, Scarborough
Printed in Great Britain by Biddles Limited, Guildford and Kings Lynn

To my father, Norman, who never reached his old age; to my mother, Doris, who continually demonstrates the creativity and resilience of older people; and to Tom, Anna, Sarah and Michael.

Grow old along with me
The best is yet to be.
      Robert Browning

Contents

Series editor's preface

The main aim of the 'Rethinking Ageing' series is to fill the gap between what we now know about older people and ageing populations as a consequence of the considerable expansion of gerontological research in the last two decades, and the relatively limited amount of knowledge which is accessible and readily available to professional and voluntary workers and others involved with older people. In addition, the series has focused on major topics in ageing of current concern or interest to that audience – to date these are: race and ethnicity, reminiscence, health and illness, ageism, elder abuse, and the psychology of growing old. However, these books are also proving attractive to another audience – lecturers, researchers and post-graduate students – which indicates that they are also fulfilling a need among academics for a concise and critical overview of what is currently known about important contemporary topics in gerontology.

This book is a particularly important contribution to the 'Rethinking Ageing' series. It fulfils one of the main aims of the series by being directly about the improvement of practice. The NHS and Community Care Act has presented new responsibilities, uncertainties and challenges to those in care management and practitioner roles who work with vulnerable older people. *Older People and Community Care* aims to assist managers and practitioners in meeting those challenges in a way which empowers older people. Beverley Hughes locates social and health care practice in the context of the new community care arrangements and the drive towards a market-led consumer oriented model of care. However, she takes a contrasting value position which is oriented towards seeing older people as citizens, first and foremost, rather than consumers. Her 'fundamental values', which provide a foundation for principles and practice, are personhood (older people are people first and old second), celebration (of age), and citizenship. Arising from this value position is her advocacy of a professional model, rather than an administrative model, of practice. This involves a skilled approach in direct work with older people, rather than a reductionist emphasis solely on practical service provision (something which has characterized community care and social work with older people). From this perspective, too, the care manager is a 'user empowerer', rather than an 'exploitative rationer', of services and resources.

In this comprehensive and penetrating analysis, Hughes also sets out the gerontological knowledge required for effective professional work, and examines the issues and dilemmas for care managers as well as practitioners involved in direct work with users and carers. This is not, therefore, a narrowly based discussion of practice: it situates work with older people critically in an analysis of the position of older people in society and the implications of policy for such work.

One vital feature of work with older people is assessment of their needs. It has been called the cornerstone of the new community care legislation. The Act offers the possibility that assessment practice will be improved and developed into the comprehensive 'needs-led' approach which is essential to improving the quality of life for older people. In Chapter 6, Hughes takes up this challenge to community care practitioners by putting forward a comprehensive, holistic and workable model of assessment which is illustrated with case material.

This book gives attention to age (along with race, gender and class) as a source of inequality. Hughes makes the important point that 'the skills involved in communicating with older people are essentially those required for good professional communication with adults generally, [but] with the important proviso that they must be applied within the context of an understanding of the experience of ageing and the impact of ageism'. Recognition of ageism as a source of inequality in our society is vital to a critical and reflective practice with older people.

Hughes also emphasizes the importance of knowledge of other issues which have a particular impact on older people. Accordingly, ageism, race, elder abuse, physical and mental health, and reminiscence – which have been the subjects of other books in this series – are also discussed here, but in direct relation to practice, these being some of the topics which constitute essential, or 'foundation', knowledge. This book can therefore be seen as facilitating that connection between knowledge and improved practice which is an overall objective of the 'Rethinking Ageing' series. It will also be invaluable as a resource for teachers, trainers and students who are concerned to achieve a genuinely empowering practice with older people.

Brian Gearing
School of Health and Social Welfare
The Open University

Preface

This book attempts to bring together two important contemporary concerns of managers and practitioners working with older people. First, the National Health Service and Community Care (NHSCC) Act has charged local authorities with the responsibility for implementing care in the community in collaboration and cooperation with the health service and other helping agencies in the statutory and independent sectors. Managers and practitioners in a variety of agencies are required to implement procedures for assessment and care management and to meet the needs of older people and carers in ways which provide flexibility and choice based upon user-participation. The community care arrangements are complex and demand, for many professionals, new ways of working and new skills, as well as the refinement and development of traditional practices. Not least, practitioners from different agencies will be required to exceed the boundaries of prevailing concepts and practices of multidisciplinary work to ensure the seamless integrated approach required to maintain elderly people at home in safety and with a good quality of life.

Second, however, these challenges also raise questions about the philosophy, values and principles which ought to underpin the definition of new tasks and functions. The helping professions generally have begun to recognize the importance of an understanding of different forms of social inequality to their practices. Agencies have increasingly incorporated statements about inequality into their policy frameworks. However, much of the interest has focused on race and gender, and to a lesser extent social class, as primary sources of inequality and discrimination. There has been much less professional attention given to old age and the need to develop anti-ageist policies and practices. This book addresses both of these important themes.

The agenda is two-fold: first, to collate and discuss the knowledge base and value base essential for the development of anti-discriminatory practice within the community care context; second, to begin to translate knowledge and values into practice and to identify the skills, approaches and awareness which anti-ageist practitioners and managers should incorporate into their work.

The structure of the book reflects this agenda. First, the Introduction discusses the principles and machinery of the NHSCC Act. Part I then deals with the foundation blocks of fundamental knowledge and values. Chapters 1 and 2 discuss theories of ageing and the facts about older people's lives. Chapter 3 sets out the essential value base for an anti-ageist approach. Part II attempts to synthesize knowledge and values with practice, identify the skills, issues and dilemmas inherent in some of the core tasks of the helping process: professional communication (Chapter 4); assessment (Chapter 5); implementing and managing care (Chapter 6); direct therapeutic work (Chapter 7); and protection (Chapter 8). Chapter 9 draws together the themes of the book and proposes a model for the conceptualization of anti-discriminatory practice in community care.

Acknowledgements

I would like to thank Oxford University Press for their kind permission to reproduce in Chapter 5 a revised version of part of an article which first appeared in the *British Journal of Social Work*, **23**(4), 1993. My grateful thanks also go to a small army of competent women who have helped me enormously with this project: Jacinta Evans and Jo Campling, for their encouragement; Jackie Boardman, Debbie McDonald, Theresa Byrne and Ruth Carter for their typing and presentation skills, and endless patience.

Introduction: Understanding the NHS and Community Care Act

The concept of community care has been a recurring theme in the post-war debate about the development of welfare. However, it is arguable that the White Paper, *Caring for People* (DoH 1989a), and the subsequent National Health Service and Community Care Act (NHSCC) (1990), constituted the first significant attempt to introduce a coherent legislative framework and a planned programme of implementation which not only married financial and organizational arrangements with a number of key political objectives, but also embraced all groups of adult service users and carers. This is not to imply that central government had at the outset a detailed grand plan. The delay in commenting upon the Griffiths Report (1988) was an indication that some of its proposals were rather unpalatable to government, not least the recommendation that local authorities were best placed to oversee a new community care initiative. Nonetheless, the resultant Act and its implementation arrangements, evolutionary though they may be, must be regarded as a watershed in the development of welfare policy and, consequently, the major determinant of both the shape of services for older people and the context and philosophy within which those services are provided.

Contingent upon the community care arrangements are changes in the roles of local authorities, developments in the nature of the economy of welfare and the balance between different sectors in that economy, as well as consequent implications for the roles of practitioners. However, while the *direction* defined by the legislation is clear in its intentions, the *outcome* in terms of key criteria, such as greater user choice and empowerment, is far from axiomatic. This is partly because the legislation embodies a number of different political objectives:

- the control of finance and resources;
- the improvement of services and extension of choice;

- changing the role of local authorities;
- a reduction in public sector provision.

It has been assumed by central government that these different objectives are mutually compatible. However, the detailed arrangements which have proved necessary to try and secure each of these objectives may eventually turn out to be *contradictory*, with success in one objective jeopardizing the achievement of another. For example, a reduction in public sector provision may not result in an extension of user choice unless a greater range of service options is developed in the voluntary and private sectors. This chapter will first examine the political origins of the legislation and attempt to unravel the diverse strands of the political agenda of which community care has become a part. Second, the substance of the legislation will be described and, third, the detailed mechanics of implementation will be examined. Finally, the implications for practitioners of the new arrangements and their relationship to the development of anti-discriminatory practice will be discussed.

The political origins of community care

The NHSCC Act emerged when it did for a variety of reasons, although the convergence of three important trends during the 1980s was probably the most important significant factor:

- Community care presented itself as another arena of social provision into which central government could extend its over-arching policy of marketization and development of private and independent providers.
- Joint policy and planning arrangements at local and central government levels had failed to develop community-based services that were adequate either in terms of the level of provision or the degree of coordination required.
- The policy of funding private residential and home nursing home care through the Department of Social Security (DSS) had not only resulted in a dramatic escalation of spending, but also in a very large and rapid rise in the number of private care homes. Consequently, many elderly people entered institutional care who could have remained in their own homes if alternative support services had been available.

These three trends are examined in more detail below.

First, one of the main planks of central government policy throughout the 1980s was the introduction of the principles and mechanics of the market into the public sector. Reforms in education and the health service, for example, created a quasi-market with internal commissioning and provider roles to simulate the buying and selling of in-house services. At the same time, new legislation required local authorities to embark upon a phased programme, determined by central government, through which many of its services had to be subjected to compulsory competitive tendering, with the aim of reducing the role of local authorities and stimulating instead the private sector. The value which underpins all of these policy initiatives is a belief that a competitive market and a mixed economy of provision will inevitably tend to provide better, cheaper services than a protected and bureaucratic public sector.

After education, social services is the highest revenue spending department for most local authorities, and within social services budgets at that time, residential and domiciliary services for elderly people consumed the largest single amount. Thus, community care for elderly people in particular presented itself to government, in both financial and policy terms, as an obvious area of provision into which market principles could and should be introduced.

Second, at local levels throughout the 1960s and 1970s, social service departments and health authorities were responsible for joint planning and service development and charged with the need to provide community-based services as alternatives to institutional care. Relatively modest amounts of joint finance were provided to promote the development of innovating projects through which to develop templates of integrated, multidisciplinary community services. However, joint planning arrangements failed to achieve those objectives and were criticized as bureaucratic and pedestrian (Working Party on Joint Planning 1985). Community care services were limited, inflexible and uncoordinated, with many users unable to obtain the services they needed, while others continued for years with a constant level of service without any subsequent review of need. In the context of growing concern about the numbers of frail elderly people likely to need support, the perceived 'problem' of elderly people became a general theme in government thinking and the need to improve joint planning as an essential prerequisite to improved services was widely recognized.

Third, however, in the early 1980s the new Conservative government had begun its long-term policy of privatizing public services. One strand within its early programme was the decision to enable people to enter private residential or nursing homes through a system of social security financing quite separate from that of local and health authorities. In the absence of a wide array of community-based services to support people at home, vast numbers of elderly people took the only option available to them and, in the face of increasing disability, entered private residential and nursing care at the expense of the public purse. This policy therefore essentially channelled public funds into the private institutional sector while leaving the domiciliary sector underdeveloped. As such, it constituted a 'perverse incentive' (Wistow *et al.* 1994: 4) that undermined the general commitment to community-based care. Private residential and nursing homes flourished and, in the absence of alternative community services, elderly people had little choice other than the decision about which home they might enter.

Strong criticism from the Audit Commission (1986) initiated a process which led to the establishment of a commission headed by Sir Roy Griffiths, whose previous advice to the then Prime Minister Thatcher had introduced market principles into the planning and delivery of health care. Widely expected to recommend that all community care services be managed by a joint health–social services board if not by the health service alone, Griffiths instead proposed that local authorities were best placed to oversee the planning and delivery of community care, with the caveat that all other relevant agencies as well as users and carers were also involved in the process.

The development of the legislation

While the tortuous route of community care development in its various forms can be traced back, at least, to the 1980s, the specific milestones which led to the NHSCC Act appeared from the end of 1980s onwards:

1985   Working Party on Joint Planning, *Progress in Partnership*
1985   House of Commons Social Services Select Committee Report, *Community Care*
1986   Audit Commission, *Making Reality of Community Care*
1987   Firth Report, *Public Support for Residential Care*
1987   National Audit Office, *Community Care Developments*
1988   Griffiths Report, *Community Care, Agenda for Action*
1989   White Paper, *Caring for People*
1990   NHSCC Act

The House of Commons Select Committee Report and, in particular, the Audit Commission Report, were critically important in their influence on the developments which were to follow. Their significance was derived in part because of the independent nature of their authorships: they stood as objective non-partisan commentaries on the state of current arrangements. However, as such, they were not restricted to an examination of how to make current policy work better. They were also able to examine the efficacy of policy itself and it was the critique of current policy, especially by the Audit Commission, which central government could not be seen to ignore. Thus, the commission re-evaluated the reasons behind the failure of community care and concluded that the primary responsibility lay not so much with the failure of joint planning at local level, but with central government policy itself. Furthermore, the strength of the report lay in the detailed marshalling of evidence to support the case, to the extent that the argument that policy had failed was established unequivocally at this point and did not have to be re-established later by Griffiths (1988).

The commission identified a number of key problems with current policy and its impact on community care development (adapted from Wistow *et al.* 1994: 4):

- the perverse financial incentive which supported the development of private institutional care at the expense of community care, through the income support system;
- lack of incentives for local authorities to develop community care options;
- the lack of a coherent policy framework within which inter-agency collaboration could develop;
- the absence of clear procedural and financial arrangements to facilitate the resettlement in the community of long-stay hospital patients;
- the lack of a systematic approach to assessment, formulating care arrangements and costing different options.

The conclusions of the commission were expressed in uncomprising terms and warned of the dire consequences of failure to act. In particular, it advocated the need for an urgent authoritative review, to which the government responded with the appointment of Sir Roy Griffiths as head of an enquiry into community care commissioned by the then Secretary of State, Norman Fowler. His remit focused upon the way in which resources could be used, rather than their overall adequacy or otherwise, and he was asked:

> . . . to review the way in which public funds are used to support community care policy and to advise [the Secretary of State] on the options for action which would improve the use of these funds as a contribution to more effective community care.
>
> (DHSS 1986)

However, Griffiths did not allow this brief to preclude him from commenting upon the need for policy objectives to be matched with adequate funding. Policy without resources, he argued, 'is the worst of all possible worlds' (Hunter and Judge 1988: 4). Griffiths began his enquiry on the basis of two important assumptions – that government had to take community care more seriously and that the underlying cause of current problems was a policy failure at national government level. In so doing, he used the review to build upon, rather than reconstruct, the conclusions of the Audit Commission. Thus, he behaved as if everyone, including government ministers, were unanimously agreed that *something had to be done* and that government had to take the initiative.

The report identified three key objectives for a new community care policy:

- *A focus upon the individual user and carer* – meeting need, improving choice, promoting self-determination. The user as consumer entered the language of community care.
- *Promotion of non-institutional support services* – to be delivered in the domestic environment and community settings to allow people to remain in their own homes.
- *A more effective targeting of resources* – to ensure those most in need received services and to avoid duplication and waste.

Griffiths (1988) emphasized in his report that his recommendations were a starting point for action, not a blueprint for implementation. In particular, a number of essential developments needed to take place before new arrangements could come to fruition. There would be a need for detailed implementation guidance, considerable extension of information systems about both need and the effective use of resources, and the inculcation of a new managerial approach within local authorities. His key recommendations included:

- the need for a clear strategic role for central government;
- the overall responsibility for development and implementation to be vested in local authorities;
- a changed role for local authorities from providing to enabling;
- a structure for effective collaboration at local level;
- new methods of financing community care;
- a one-door approach to publically funded residential and nursing home care;
- the development of a mixed economy of care;

- the stimulation, through financial mechanisms, of greater diversity of services, particularly in the voluntary and private sectors;
- designation of specific responsibility for community care to a minister of state with proper support for development and implementation.

The responsibility for, and oversight of, community care vested in local authorities was tempered with the recommendation that the role of local authorities should change. Rather than providing services directly, local authorities should become planners, commissioners and enablers, ensuring adequate services are provided but largely by other agents:

> The primary function of the public services is to design and arrange the provision of care and support in line with people's needs. That care and support can be provided from a variety of sources. There is value in a multiplicity of provision, not least from the consumer's point of view, because of the widening of choice, flexibility, innovation and competition it should stimulate. The proposals are therefore aimed at stimulating the further development of the 'mixed economy' of care. It is vital that social services authorities should see themselves as arrangers and purchasers of care services – not as monopolistic providers.
>
> (Griffiths Report 1988: para. 3.4)

The concept of the enabling role at the macro level of the strategic local authority was also mirrored at the micro level of the user–practitioner relationship, with the recommendation that the professional worker acting on behalf of the local authority should adopt a 'case management' approach: assessing need with the user, defining a suitable package of care and purchasing the constituent services on behalf of the user/carer. Perhaps one of the most radical proposals was that concerning the public finance of residential and nursing home care. Griffiths argued that all applications for assistance should be subject to assessment of need, and income and finance should be administered by the same body – the local authority.

The White Paper which followed in November 1989 accepted most of the Griffiths proposals and endorsed the three basic tenets of user choice, promoting non-institutional services and targeting. Its six key objectives for service delivery were:

- to promote the development of domiciliary, day and respite services to enable people to live in their own homes whenever feasible and sensible;
- to ensure that service providers make practical support for carers a high priority;
- to make proper assessment of need and good case management the cornerstone of high quality care;
- to promote the development of a flourishing independent sector alongside good quality public services;
- to clarify the responsibilities of agencies and so make it easier to hold them to account for their performance;
- to secure better value for taxpayers' money by introducing a new funding structure for social care.

(DoH 1989a: 5)

However, while the new framework for organizing and developing care, and thereby ensuring the key outcomes for users, was largely based on the Griffiths recommendations, a crucial element was missing: the diversion of money from the social security budget to the local authorities was not to be ringfenced for community care in the long term as Griffiths had advocated. A specific grant was to be diverted to local authorities in order to implement the outcomes of individual assessment and stimulate the development of services in the private and voluntary sectors, but receipt of the grant was conditional upon the publication of satisfactory collaborative community care plans and would be ringfenced only in the short term.

Equally significant as the objectives themselves were the organizational arrangements defined for achieving them, and it is through the means of implementation that the government succeeded in using community care as another vehicle for its more fundamental policy of marketization of the public sector. The organizational arrangements included:

- The requirement that local authorities demonstrate not only that *planning* services involves collaboration with other key agents such as voluntary agencies, health authorities and user/carer groups, but also that the *outcomes* are achieved collaboratively.
- The organization of service delivery to users and carers through a systematic process of assessment and case management, including devolved budgets and decentralized purchasing.
- The separation of purchaser and provider functions at all levels in the organization – operational, managerial and strategic – in order to simulate not only market relations between the local authorities and the providers, but also an internal market within social services authorities themselves.

Thus, a contract culture was to be applied to the provision of personal social services and social services departments would need to develop the abilities to specify, commission and monitor services delivered by other agencies. The promotion of a mixed economy of care was to be achieved by the authorities:

- determining clear specifications of service requirements, and arrangements for tenders and contracts;
- taking steps to stimulate the development of private and not-for-profit agencies;
- identifying areas of their work which are sufficiently self-contained to be suitable for 'floating-off' as self-managing units;
- stimulating the development of a new voluntary sector.

(DoH 1989a: 23)

The process by which these new arrangements and diverse objectives were to fit together is inevitably complex, so much so that immediately after the NHSCC Bill was enacted in June 1990, the government announced that implementation would be phased between April 1991 and April 1993, beginning with the establishment of inspection units and complaints procedures, the transfer of specific grants for mental illness and drugs/alcohol services, and the early development of the organizational systems needed for full implementation. By April 1993, local authorities were required to be ready

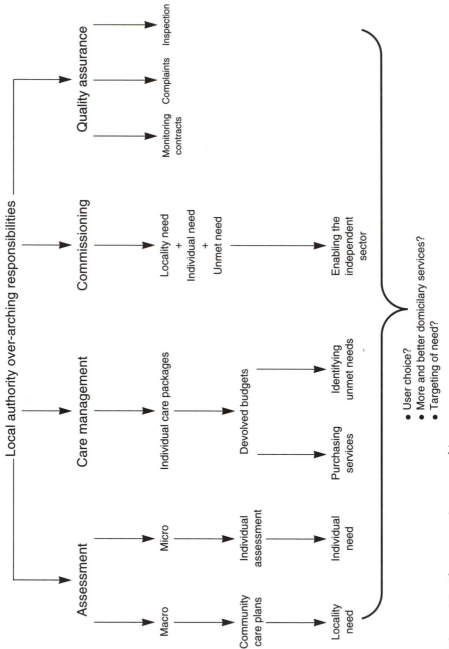

Figure 0.1 The community care machinery

for all new cases and the application of assessment and case management systems, drawing upon services identified in community care plans and provided by a growing independent sector.

The community care machinery

Figure 1 represents the key elements within the local authorities' over-arching responsibilities and describes the way in which these elements are connected, at least theoretically, to promote the overall outcomes of user/carer choice, stimulation of domiciliary independent sector services and the targeting of need. There are four key cogs to the community care machinery. These are interconnected and together are meant to drive the process: assessment, care management, commissioning and quality assurance.

1 Assessment of need at both the 'macro' level of the locality and the 'micro' level of the individual user/carer is fundamental to the process. At the macro level, the local authority is required to gather information to enable it to form a comprehensive picture of the current and likely future needs within the adult population for community care services, and to use that information to produce, along with other key agents, a community care plan to define the direction for service development. The community care plan is the basic blueprint for each authority and its partners for the implementation and evolution of community care in its area, and ought to be, therefore, the key policy document which informs the planning and purchasing of services at the strategic level.

Assessment at the level of the individual user or carer is equally fundamental and the government has stated clearly that this should be an assessment of *need*, taking 'account of the wishes of the individual and his or her carer, and of the carer's ability to provide care, and where possible should include their active participation' (DoH 1989a: 19). Assessment should not focus specifically on the user's suitability or eligibility for a particular service but, especially when needs are multiple or complex, should involve a comprehensive, multidisciplinary and holistic examination of the person's strengths, weaknesses, needs and resources in the round.

Assessment at the macro level and the summation of individual assessments, including information about unmet need, over a period of time should produce information essential to two other elements in the system: care management and commissioning.

2 Care management takes place at the micro level and involves the implementation of a package of services, which together will meet as far as possible the needs defined in the individual user/carer assessment. Care management thus differs from assessment in that it must inevitably take place in the context of available resources, and care managers must have some degree of responsibility for, or at least knowledge of, the budget available for the purchase of service within a given period of time. The extent to which organizational arrangements will include a degree of devolution of budgets down to care managers varies across different local authorities.

In addition to purchasing services to supply individual care packages, it is also important that care managers collate information about assessed need which cannot be met, either because the budget is not sufficient or because appropriate services are not yet available for purchase. The care manager, then, is to:

> . . . take responsibility for ensuring that individuals needs are regularly reviewed, resources are effectively managed and that each service user has a single point of contact. The 'care manager' will then be employed by the social services authority but this need not always be so. He or she may or may not be the designated person responsible for the original assessment and design stages.
>
> (DoH 1989a: 21)

Both the Griffiths Report and the White Paper refer to this role as *case* management. Later guidance transmuted the term to *care* management and it has been suggested that the change illustrates the lack of understanding at government level about the implications of the role for practitioners and managers (Huxley 1993). This issue is discussed more fully in Chapter 6.

3 Commissioning. The commissioning role of the local authority is the mechanism which connects the public, voluntary and private sectors and is the means by which the government envisages the mixed economy of care will be catalysed. The local authority must spend, under current arrangements, 85 per cent of the special transitional grant (the money divested from the Department of Social Security to social services departments) in the private and voluntary sectors, to purchase services which care managers can then draw upon for care packages. The 85 per cent rule thus ensures that local authorities cannot use the grant to develop in-house services but rather to stimulate the independent sector. Thus, the *commissioning role*, in government parlance, tranforms the local authority into an *enabling* authority, using its financial resources to kick-start local non-statutory agencies into developing services to meet local need.

The definition of local need should emerge from the outcome of the assessment and care management processes:

Local need = Locality need + Individual needs + Unmet need
↓	↓	↓
Outcome of	Summation of	Outcome of
macro	micro	case
assessment	assessments	management

Thus, assessment and care management are not only key processes at the level of user–practitioner relationships. They are also vital elements in the strategic forward-planning and commissioning processes through which, over time, the market of care moves closer to providing services to match local need.

Quite how the commissioning process and contract culture will evolve remains unclear, as in the first year or so of implementation most local authorities have been unable to spend all their transitional grant in the independent sector, which has been both slow to respond and, in the case of voluntary agencies, wary about moving from a 'grant-aided' to a 'contract-for-services' basis of financial support. The change implies, in future, a different relationship between local authorities and voluntary agencies, who are also aware of the potential threat posed by contracts not only to their financial stability, but also to their power to innovate and challenge.

For local authorities, on the other hand, holding the purse-strings ought to carry with it the power of the purchaser to determine not only what the 'market' provides, but also its quality and price. In practice, however, authorities have found this power has existed more in theory than in practice, as the market has shown itself to be an imperfect mechanism for ensuring the provision of care for vulnerable or dependent individuals. For example, continuity of provision is an important criterion for many users. Thus, the decision to switch contracts is not as simple as it might be, for example, if the authority were purchasing commodities rather than, say, bathing services. Furthermore, as grant aid to voluntary agencies has diminished, contracts have been used to support voluntary agencies financially without the rigorous specification of service that contracting should involve. Indeed, as Flynn and Common (1990) have found, the close relationship which exists between individuals in the local authority and voluntary agencies, while facilitating the contracting process, may also jeopardize the strict definition of standards and impartial monitoring and evaluation.

Wistow *et al.* (1994) identify the two competing concepts of the enabling authority: the 'competitive council' and the 'community government'. The former derives from New Right critiques of the public sector as inherently bureaucratic, monolithic, high-spending and unaccountable. It employs the concept of the enabling authority as the banner under which the role is reduced to that of specification and awarding of contracts. It is a 'minimalist view of local government' (Clarke and Stewart 1990: 5), both in terms of the people employed (purchasers not providers) and the technocratic, administrative jobs they are expected to perform (specification, inviting tenders, monitoring contracts). The community government model, by contrast, defines enabling in a much broader way, embracing the idea of local authorities working with local people to define and meet needs. Contracting with outside bodies is not precluded but, rather than being the driving force behind the authority's role and actions, becomes instead just one of a number of means by which the authority fulfils its enabling responsibility to the community (Clarke and Stewart 1990).

4 *Quality assurance*. The final cog in the chain is the duty to assure the quality of services provided whether by the authority or contracted agencies. There are three mechanisms which address quality assurance: complaints procedures, inspection and contract monitoring. All authorities are required to establish and publish procedures by which users and carers can complain about services they have received. However, the existence of such a procedure does not, *per se*, ensure that the user is guaranteed redress or satisfaction. Many complaints are concerned with the level of service or charges and, as such, can only be met by a change in policy by local politicians. It is crucial, therefore, that managers and councillors receive periodically a detailed analysis of complaints over a period of time, in order to evaluate not only whether the procedure itself is accessible and effective, but also whether the outcomes of complaints suggest that certain aspects of policy or resource allocation warrant re-examination.

Inspections units must be established, at arms length from the social service directorate, and should initially be 'charged with inspecting and reporting on both local authority and registerable independent residential care homes' (DoH 1989a: 45). The role of the units, however, is evolving to include inspection of other services and in many authorities they have also become the home of the complaints procedure.

Monitoring and evaluating contracts is a crucial element in the contracting process. Authorities have not been given resources to execute this function and yet the processes of specification and monitoring are both time-consuming and labour-intensive, as compulsory competitive tendering for other services has already demonstrated. Furthermore, the criteria for monitoring and evaluation are problematic when the services in question are a form of personal care. How far should user satisfaction be the primary criterion? What are the constraints on users/carers expressing dissatisfaction with a service upon which they are dependent? What should be the balance between subjective and objective criteria? Contract monitoring and evaluation, if implemented properly, involves all the dilemmas and expertise of qualitative and quantitive research, of which local authority personnel have had little experience and for which they are not trained.

Implications for practitioners: Community care and anti-discriminatory practice

It remains to be seen how far the community care machinery will produce the outcomes of greater user choice, more flexible and better quality domiciliary services with more efficient targeting on those most in need. The machinery, as designed, has an internal rational coherence which, theoretically, ought to mean that the elements work together smoothly, each connected to the other and together providing a driving force for change.

The principles of an anti-discriminatory approach, as I shall discuss later, underline the importance of participation, choice, integration and normalization. The community care machinery, in itself, is not unsympathetic to such principles and could be utilized to foster anti-discriminatory practice. What is important is not the machinery itself but the *values* which define the way it operates and the consequent implications both for users/carers and the roles of practitioners. The values which underpin the government's approach define users and carers as consumers (but does not give them any direct purchasing power), local authorities as strategic planners and administrators of contracts, the competitive market as the vehicle for pluralism and quality, and the practitioner as the interface between the user and the market. The detailed implementation of this concept may also tend to define services in simple, practical ways and reduce the scope for professional practice with more complex issues involving, for example, emotional problems, conflicts of interest, conflict, moral dilemma or loss.

However, a different set of underpinning values would set the machinery off in a rather different direction: user as citizen, with implied rights rather than just purchasing power; local authorities as guardians of community aspirations; partnership between key stakeholders as the model for planning and development; continuity between assessor and service provider roles for professonals; therapeutic as well as practical services for users/carers. The language of community care has been couched in terms which suggest its aims are consistent with those of anti-discrimination. However, the underlying values of the prescribed model raise legitimate questions about how far anti-discriminatory principles can be achieved in practice. These issues will be examined in further detail in the final chapter.

PART I

Knowledge and values

1

Theories of ageing

Why is theory important?

It is not accidental that a book which is essentially about *practice* begins with a discussion of *theory*. Theories – ideas, frameworks for understanding, hypotheses, speculations, values, explanations – form the basis of all activities in our personal and professional lives. *Actions* do not arise out of an ideological vacuum. However deeply embedded they may be, ideas, beliefs, values and knowledge (i.e. theories) are the mainspring of behaviour, the reasons why we do the things we do. Theory, therefore, is essential to understanding both ourselves and the people around us.

However, in the professional arena, theory is particularly important for several reasons. First, social and health care workers are powerful. They make assessments, recommendations and decisions which affect profoundly the lives of other people. On what bases are these professional judgements made? How can they be accounted for? How can they be evaluated? If a professional worker judges that Mrs Smith, aged 84 years, is 'at risk' or 'not at risk', that judgement cannot be made without implicit or explicit reference to knowledge and theory. The 'facts' about Mrs Smith cannot themselves lead to the judgement. Rather, the facts have to be located and evaluated within the context of all available knowledge and theory about old people in general, about old women in particular, about cultural identity and family relations, about risk and its circumstances. Unless the knowledge and theory being used are made explicit, the validity of the professional judgement cannot be questioned and the outcomes arising from that judgement cannot subsequently be evaluated.

The second reason, however, concerns the nature of theory itself. Unlike scientific theory, theories about human beings and their social situations are not 'objective' and value free. Theories at all levels in the human sciences are

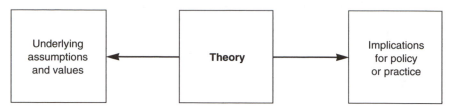

Figure 1.1   Values, theory and action

based on some fundamental assumptions or values which have to be made explicit (Howe 1987). Furthermore, different theories lead policy-makers and professionals in quite different directions in terms of what, if anything, needs to be done (Fig. 1.1).

For example, a comparison of a biological theory of ageing to a sociological approach illustrates this point. A biologist may understand ageing and the condition and experience of old people largely in terms of a predetermined pattern controlled by genetic endowment and biological processes of decline. The underlying assumption underpinning that approach is a view of human beings as biologically *determined*, with little scope for the influence of non-biological factors. This might lead policy-makers and practitioners to concentrate on developing and targeting services to support or care for very dependent old people rather than identifying any means by which dependency could be prevented or reduced. A sociologist, on the other hand, might see the condition and experience of old people primarily as the result of social and economic factors, and attitudes to old people in particular cultures. The underlying assumption here is that the human condition is flexible and adaptable to social forces. Thus, the implications for policy and practice address the need to alter the social, economic and political conditions which shape old people's lives.

It is important to understand that different theories offer different *levels* of understanding, particularly in relation to human circumstances and human behaviour within any given society or culture. At the macro level, for example, theories attempt to make sense of the broad characteristics of elderly people as a group. Within this macro level of theory there will, nevertheless, be competing perspectives, each offering a different way of understanding the same observed phenomenon and each emphasizing different factors as the key explanations. At this level, theories propound a particular view of old age within its societal context – that is, they *construct* an image of old age. The images created by the various theoretical perspectives – biological, psychologi-cal, sociological, political-economic – are intrinsically different and create quite distinct pictures of the experience and social condition of older people. However, as practitioners and people interested in understanding and helping older people, we also need a range of theories at the 'micro' level to help us make sense of the particular situation of an individual older person. At this level, we might need to draw upon theories of gender and race and how these factors interact with old age; knowledge and theory about mental health, family dynamics, systems theory or crisis intervention. We need to apply and utilize a range of knowledge and theory to make assessments of individualized situations and to identify strategies for addressing problems or needs.

Finally, we will also need to use theories at the 'interactional' level in order both to understand the behaviour of a particular individual and to inform the way we behave as practitioners towards the people with whom we work. At this level, then, we need to be aware of and apply theories of communication, counselling, understanding verbal and non-verbal behaviour, feelings and reactions, different techniques (and their underlying theoretical premises) for helping people express themselves and change. Later chapters in this book address theories at the micro and interactional levels. However, this chapter is concerned with mapping the broad panoramas created by competing perspectives at the macro level, identifying the values and assumptions upon which each is based and establishing the theoretical framework for the remainder of this book.

'Macro' theories of ageing: Gerontology

Within the social and human sciences, the relationships between fact, theory and value, at the macro level, are not straightforward. Theory is often built upon fundamental and essentially untestable assumptions and values. Specific theories can hold such sway for a time that their propositions become elevated to the status of unquestioned 'facts', upon which policy and practice is predicated. As one notable gerontologist has contended, 'facts are inseparable from our "perceptual filters"' (Hendricks 1992: 32). Nowhere is this more graphically illustrated than in the historical development of theories of ageing, or gerontology. Gerontology has a number of streams within each of which different perspectives are discernible: biological, psychological and social. The typology which follows is inevitably somewhat personal, with particular groupings, inclusions and omissions which may differ from those of other commentators. However, the intention is to provide a broad view of competing perspectives within gerontology and to illuminate the underlying assumptions upon which each is based.

Biological gerontology

Biological or biomedical perspectives have generally focused upon the search for the reasons why and how human beings change over time in terms of their biological and physiological characteristics. A key question, the answer to which remains unresolved between the different schools of thought, is whether or not there exists a normal, unpathological process of ageing or whether ageing, by its very biological nature, is existentially a pathological process involving loss of capacity and, ultimately, the demise of the human organism itself. Indeed, biological theorists have not yet agreed upon a definition of what human ageing *is*.

Bromley (1988: 30) suggests that 'human ageing can be conveniently defined as a complex, cumulative, time-related process of psychobiological deterioration occupying the post-development (adult) phase of life'. Thus, he adopts the view that ageing is an intrinsically degenerative process that begins as soon as a person has reached the peak of functional capacity which, in terms of basic biological characteristics such as skeleton size, muscular strength, cardiac output or basal metabolic rate, is around 18–25 years of age. Adult ageing, from then on, is viewed as a summation of pathological conditions:

> One way to conceptualise the course of human life is to think of it as following a trajectory in which the individual is launched at conception and reaches a maximum level of functional capacity or vitality in early adult life. From then on, because of intrinsic 'design' faults and extrusive damage, functional vitality decreases gradually, or at times abruptly, until the individual is no longer capable of coping with the demands of life, and dies.
>
> (Bromley 1988: 25)

An alternative biological perspective, however, postulates the existence of a normal ageing process which, at least hypothetically, would characterize the biological changes which would take place if illness or disease did not intervene. However, this normal process – or senescence as it is called by biologists – is one of increasing inefficiency in the functioning of the organism, decreasing survival capacity and diminishing ability to adapt (Victor 1994). Thus, even when conceptualized as a natural, normal (i.e. a non-pathological) process, ageing is characterized as essentially degenerative in biological terms.

In practice, the distinction between these two perspectives has been blurred and it is often unclear what can or should be regarded as a 'normal' consequence of the ageing process, and what should be regarded as pathological, a disease. For example, it is a common view among general practitioners and lay people alike that certain chronic diseases are almost inevitable in old age and therefore have to be borne rather than remedied. Arthritis or dementia, for example, are quite incorrectly regarded as part and parcel of growing old, and this view is an example of the pejorative construction of old age to which, to some extent, biological perspectives have contributed. This is clearly exemplified by Strehler's (1962) attempt to define ageing more precisely and to distinguish ageing from other biological processes. In so doing, four criteria of the process of ageing were identified:

- *Universality* – the process must happen to every person.
- *Internality* – the processes must be initiated from within the organism and not by some external hazard or consequence of lifestyle.
- *Progressiveness* – the processes occur gradually, over time and the effects are cumulative.
- *Degeneration* – the processes must have a harmful effect on the person.

Thus Strehler (1962) explicitly defines ageing as harmful, not developmental, and thereby excludes from the definition of ageing any potential for the individual to develop capacities in some areas of life, or to adapt capacities to new biological or environmental circumstances.

A number of biological theories have attempted to explain why human organisms change biologically as they age:

- *Programmed cellular activity.* Human cells are thought to have a pre-programmed fixed life and a self-generative capacity that decreases with age. Thus, as a person ages, so the capacity of cells to reproduce decreases, and the time taken to reproduce increases, resulting in a gradual loss of functional abilities. However, while laboratory experiments involving cell division rates have shown that cells from young people divide more quickly and efficiently than those from older people, they have not yet shown any consistent differences between men and women of similar ages. And yet the life expectancy of women is higher than that of men – a phenomenon for which, therefore, there seems to be no *biological* basis, but which has to be explained entirely by social and other factors. If life expectancy differences cannot be explained biologically, to what extent, then, can biological processes be the primary factor in life expectancy, and therefore, ageing *per se*?
- *Mutation consequences.* As cells divide, errors and unprogrammed mutations occur, producing cells not designed, and therefore less efficient, for sustaining the functional activities essential to life.
- *Immune system activity.* The immune system produces antibodies in response to invading cells or organisms. However, these antigens themselves are thought to catalyse ageing changes, as a by-product to their immune response activity. An alternative hypothesis of this theme is the possibility that errors arising from the immune response fail to distinguish between healthy and hazardous cells, fail to eradicate hazardous cells and thereby result in a less efficient level of functioning.

It is clear that from birth to, say, the age of 80 years, human beings undergo bodily and functional changes. As a person advances towards old age, a range of biological consequences can be observed, including changes to skin conditions, hair, muscular ability, respiratory ability, cardiac function, meta-bolic and gastrointestinal systems and the activity rates of various organs (Briggs 1990). However, the biological perspective does not appear to take account of the way in which many individuals *adapt* to those changes, nor to the potential for development in other non-biological abilities. For example, to what extent does *experience* counteract the consequences of diminishing functional abilities? How far do attributes such as creativity, skills, adaptability, decision-making, risk-taking or learning depend more upon psychological attitudes, economic resources or personal experience and less upon the level of biological functioning at any particular point in time?

While important in identifying the changes which may impinge on individuals as they age, albeit at different rates and to different degrees, biological theories have contributed to an unnecessarily negative and there-fore discriminatory image of old people, and have to some extent been the theoretical legitimation for the essentially ageist view that old people are a burden upon their families and on society (MacIntyre 1977; Hickey 1992). This is not to argue that biological knowledge and theory has no place in the armoury of the would-be helper. Knowledge about biological ageing is an essential backcloth against which the circumstances facing an individual older person must be understood. However, as a theoretical framework for understanding the experience of ageing – what it is like to be an old human body – it is in fact extremely oppressive, as the testimonies of many older people indicate (e.g. Hemmings 1985; Ford and Sinclair 1987). Nevertheless, perhaps because of their apparent scientific objectivity, biological perspectives have dominated the study and research of ageing, and the implicit view of ageing as negative and degenerative has been the basis of social and economic policies, as well as attitudes, to older people for many years. As Bytheway and Johnson (1990: 31) summarize:

> The indisputable and visible evidence of change over time is interpreted as evidence of decline and has permeated every approach to ageing . . . The social responses to old people are rooted in the biological model of decline.

Psychological gerontology

For some considerable time during its own evolution as a discipline, the subjects of ageing and older people were noticeable within psychology only by their absence. For many years, the Freudian view prevailed – that is, older people have characters and personalities which are rigidly structured and not amenable to development or change (Knight 1986). Psychological perspectives of all varieties have been much more concerned with understanding childhood and child development, and the behaviour of younger people generally, than illuminating the process of ageing from a psychological perspective. When psychology did begin to address the process of ageing, its early hypotheses – like its biological counterparts – tended to focus on perceived decline in psychological well-being and adaptive ability as individuals enter later life. The implicit concept was that psychological human functioning followed the biological trajectory of rapid, positive development in early life, reaching a peak in early adulthood, followed by inevitable decline and increasing loss of function towards old age. Experimental, or clinical, psychology appeared to confirm this view with research data which suggested, for example, that the ability to learn new skills took longer for older people, that memory and recall was less efficient, response rate was slower and that cognitive functioning in general declined in old age. However, much of this research used a design which compared the functioning of older people with that of a group of contemporary young people and thus made no allowance for the impact of different socio-economic factors or different life experiences of people in these two age cohorts. Nevertheless, data which in effect were comparing the performances of two very different groups of people, whose different experiences probably had a significant impact on their levels of performance, were used to suggest, therefore, that the psychological performance of any given individual will change through time. Results which may have been produced by the effect of using different cohorts were thus attributed to the effects of ageing itself. Subsequent work has not only challenged the validity of this methodology, taking no account, as it does, of social and other environmental factors in explaining cohort differences, but has also produced results on learning which counter earlier findings. Experiments on the acquisition of new skills suggest, for example, that while older workers may take more time and be initially less confident than younger people in learning new techniques, they subsequently out-perform younger people in terms of accuracy, reliability and output.

Nevertheless, 'ageing as psychological decline', like its biological counterpart, has pervaded attitudes and policy towards older people and its influence is still evident (Stokes 1992; Stuart-Hamilton 1994). Many older people themselves, for example, expect their recall faculties to begin to fade as they age, attributing minor memory lapses, which in a younger person would go unnoticed, to the process of ageing or even to the onset of dementia. It is particularly evident, furthermore, that theories of psychological decline are not culturally unbiased, but have emerged within societies which have a view of old people as burdensome and problematic. This perspective does not appear to be able to encompass, for example, the belief in other societies that old age is a time of wisdom and enhanced psychological functioning, and is thus a predominantly white euro-centric perspective purporting to offer a universal theory (Clayton and Birren 1980). Furthermore, later psychologists have themselves criticized their predecessors in cognitive psychology for failing to take sufficient account of social and environmental factors as determinants of cognitive functioning. For example, Rabbitt cites the impact of living in a residential environment on the cognitive abilities of residents compared with people of similar age living in their own homes. Living in an environment which removes the need to think and organize their daily lives, residents have to delve more into their own pasts to retrieve interesting subjects for conversation:

> In this static, communal environment rehearsal of everyday minutiae makes poor conversation. When the theatre of the mind becomes the only show in town archival memories begin to be actively explored for scripts.
>
> (Rabbitt 1988: 503)

Theories which define ageing as development rather than degeneration imply a different set of assumptions and propositions. Erikson (1965) hypothesized that each individual's life progresses through a series of psychological stages, each of which involves a psychological conflict, the successful resolution of which is important in determining how the individual is able to meet the challenges and conflicts of subsequent stages of life (Table 1.1). The function of each stage is the accomplishment of particular developmental tasks

Table 1.1   Erikson's eight life stages

Developmental stage	Crisis to be resolved
Infancy	Basic trust *vs* basic mistrust
Childhood (1)	Autonomy *vs* doubt
Childhood (2)	Initiative *vs* guilt
Childhood (3)	Industry *vs* inferiority
Adolescence	Ego identity *vs* role confusion
Young adulthood	Intimacy *vs* isolation
Adulthood	Generativity *vs* stagnation
Old age	Integrity *vs* despair

After Erikson (1965).

which will be required in the next stage and later in life. Developed initially as a framework for understanding early development in life, its application to adulthood and old age was only sketchily drawn, with old age constructed somewhat vaguely as a 'summing-up' phase prior to death. Later development of the theory, however, elaborates on the importance of later stages, each of which presents the individual with its own development challenge and, thereby, the potential for growth.

While each stage is not assigned to a particular chronological age, the stages are thought to be sequential, with the outcome of the crisis at one stage influencing the experience and resolution of those which follow. In adulthood, the major task is that of 'generativity' – that is, ensuring the establishment and guidance of the next generation not only within one's own family but also at a social or political level. The conflicting state is 'stagnation', in which the individual remains centred on him or herself. The last task of life according to Erikson is the achievement of 'ego integrity', an internalized acceptance of the validity, worth and meaning of one's own life. This does not mean having to see one's life as 'successful', but rather accepting the achievements, the regrets, the failures as part and parcel of a unique and personal experience.

Life span developmental psychology has been criticized particularly in respect of its one-dimensional view of life span. Despite considerable diversity in the patterns of people's lives not only between different cultures but also *within* Western European cultures, Erikson's stages seem to imply a pattern of life which consists of childhood in a two-parent family, adolescence, marriage and producing children of one's own with a consistent partner. It reflects the conventional Western European values about what is, or should be, the normal pattern of life, even though this pattern characterizes an ever-decreasing minority of the lives of people in modern society. Nevertheless, despite its cultural relativity, life span psychology embodies three specific principles, which have been important to the development of ideas about ageing. First, old age is clearly connected, theoretically within the framework, to the course of an individual's earlier life. It is not constructed as a separate, distinct phase with qualitatively different characteristics. Thus, old people are *people*. Second, the impact of social and environmental factors is acknowledged. The extent to which a person is able to achieve resolution of a life stage crisis is contingent not only upon his or her own personal psychological characteristics, but also upon the hazards or opportunities which he or she is facing at the time. Third, because of the combined impact of self *and* environment on conflict resolution and developmental task acquisition, each individual emerges from each life stage with different degrees of success, and therefore goes forward to the next stage with different degrees of preparedness. The cumulative effect of these different outcomes results in considerable diversity between people, and this potential for diversity increases as people progress through life towards old age (Erikson *et al.* 1986). However, as a psychological approach, developmental psychology goes no further in analysing the sources of diversity, and so Erikson and subsequent commentators did not consider the impact of life factors such as gender, race, social class or disability upon the ability to negotiate life stages.

A third and more recent theme within psychology is the emergence of a strand of thinking concerned with understanding the subjective experience of ageing from a psychological perspective. This is distinct from a sociological analysis based on life biography or life history, although it touches these concepts. For example, analytic psychology is concerned with the emergence of an integrated sense of self through the process of individuation, and this task is one which is thought to predominate in the second half of life (Biggs 1993). Jung (1972) thus postulates an important and distinct psychological task for the second half of life. However, the values of modern society are such that the process of individuation is not easily accommodated. Social images of ageing and old people deny the importance or even the feasibility of development in later life. A related concept is that of continuity, which suggests that in the process of ageing, a person will attempt to continue the patterns, habits and lifestyle which have characterized earlier life (Atchley 1989). Thus, in so far as old age presents challenges to continuity through retirement, physical changes or loss, the ageing individual will respond in whatever ways enable him or her to negotiate the disadvantages and preserve continuity as far as possible. Thus, different individuals will respond in different ways and, indeed, will have different views about what is important to preserve and what can be relinquished or changed. Some of these views will be entirely idiosyncratic; some may be conditioned by earlier life history or by personal characteristics such as race or gender. Thus, the *subjective* meaning of ageing for the individual has to be understood. While these perspectives present a necessary critique to those theories which do not acknowledge diversity and implicitly define old people as a homogeneous, degenerating group, they offer a myriad of patterns of ageing from which it is difficult to extract some general themes and, therefore, as a framework for understanding, have perhaps travelled too far in the direction of individualizing personal experience.

Social gerontology

Social gerontology is the most differentiated of the three theoretical streams and is characterized by its own pattern of evolution. While social gerontology in all its forms has sought to understand elderly people and their life-worlds within a *societal* context, different generations of social gerontological theory have conceptualized the individual–societal dialectic in different ways.

Disengagement theory (Cumming and Henry 1961) is perhaps the most well known of the earliest generation of social gerontological perspectives which sought primarily to identify the individual characteristics of 'successful' ageing. Within the individual–societal dynamic, social structure was taken for granted, and only individual adaptations to that structure examined. From empirical data based on a study of fairly able and economically secure Americans aged 50–90 years, three basic tenets were postulated:

- As people age, they withdraw, or disengage, from primary roles and activities of social and economic life.
- Disengagement is a natural and personally satisfying process for the individual, releasing them from expectations and demands for which they are less and less equipped.

- Disengagement is also functional for society, releasing roles and opportunities for younger people.

Disengagement theory is a functionalist perspective, portraying the mutual withdrawal of old people and society as a process which ensures continuity of the system and equilibrium between different social groups. Successful ageing is defined as the acquiescent, tranquil acceptance of social withdrawal and the characteristics, or quality, of life which follow such withdrawal. Implicit within this perspective is the view, therefore, that old people differ from younger people in their desires, wishes and needs, especially in terms of purposeful roles, social interaction and activity. It conveys a 'rocking chair' view of old age which legitimated, on both sides of the Atlantic for many years, social and economic policies which separated old people from the rest of the population and validated a condition of 'structured dependency' (Townsend 1981). In terms of practice, it is not difficult to understand how this perspective justified the sterility of life in residential care for old people (Wilkin and Hughes 1987) or the attitude of professionals to problems of living that 'It's just your age'.

The second wave within social gerontology began not so much as a coherent theoretical challenge to disengagement theory, but from the gradual emergence into gerontological consciousness that, in fact, satisfaction with life for older people depends on the same criteria as for younger people. The evidence was gathered initially by American sociologists seeking to establish valid measures of life satisfaction through the administration of questionnaires to different groups within the population (Neugarten *et al.* 1961; Havighurst 1968). Similar exercises were also conducted in Britain (Bigot 1974; Felce and Jenkins 1978). The results demonstrated that meaningful roles, activities and relationships were equally important to satisfaction with life in old age as at younger ages. Thus, while not commenting on the social conditions which lead to withdrawal, 'activity theory' challenged the underlying assumption of disengagement theory that old people are essentially a different breed and that old age is, existentially, a qualitatively different time of life (Hughes and Wilkin 1980).

Activity theory re-attached old age to the continuum of life and reconnected old people to their own histories and to the rest of the population. In Britain, in particular, activity theory led to the introduction of structured activities in institutional settings (e.g. Lunt *et al.* 1977) and the provision of communal areas in elderly-specific housing, such as sheltered housing. However, as later developments were to suggest, well-being, morale and life satisfaction are not enhanced by such enforced or ritualistic activity, however well meaning, but by interactions and activities which are personally and socially meaningful for the individual (Gubrium 1973; Liang *et al.* 1980; Longino and Kart 1982).

The third generation of social gerontology perspectives began from the premise that ageing must be examined in the context of the society in which it takes place – its structure, history and values – and applied the conceptual and methodological tools of mainstream sociology to social gerontology (Hendricks and Leedham 1991). Subcultural approaches viewed older people as a distinct group within society and charted the economic and social distinctions between older people and the rest of society (Rose 1965; Estes 1979). In Britain, the application of a critical perspective to social gerontology began to question the inequality observed between older people, as a group, and younger people, and identified negative social attitudes and socio-economic policies as primarily responsible for the social condition of older people (Phillipson 1972; Walker 1980, 1981; Townsend 1981). Critical gerontology rejects the notion that the condition and experiences of old people derive essentially from the biological process of ageing and looks instead to the social construction of ageing under capitalism as the primary reason for the marginalization of old people.

The underlying assumption is that old age is not a period of inevitable dependency, either physically or economically. Critical gerontology thereby offers a coherent *theoretical* challenge to the assumptions underpinning disengagement theory and focuses attention not on the individual, but on the societal factors which account for individual experience:

> The critical approach argues that old age is a socially constructed experience and embodies two central principles. Firstly, it argues that the factors and criteria which define a good quality of life for older people are exactly those which apply in general terms, to people of all ages. In this respect, critical social gerontology has at last provided a theoretical challenge to disengagement theory whose legacy has persisted for so long. Secondly, the critical approach accepts that the experience of old age is determined as much by economic and social factors as by biological or individual characteristics.
>
> (Hughes 1990: 47)

However, early expositions of critical gerontology have been criticized for their failure to acknowledge the impact of individual difference on the experience of ageing and, with the exclusive focus on the structural position of older people as a group, of painting a picture of that group as homogeneous (Estes *et al.* 1992). Thus, the impact of class, gender, race, culture and life history on the experience and condition of old age was ignored (Hughes and Mtezuka 1992).

The most recent generation of social gerontological perspectives have begun to address this issue. A moral and political economy of ageing aims:

> . . . to move beyond a critique of conventional gerontology and to develop an understanding of the character and significance of variations in the treatment of the aged and to relate these to broader systemic trends. Another important task is to understand how the ageing process itself is affected by the systematic treatment and location of the aged in society.
>
> (Estes *et al.* 1984: 25)

Thus, this perspective proposes that the dependent condition of elderly people in Western society, and, indeed, the pattern of the ageing process itself, are conditioned by their location within the socio-economic structure both now, as older people, and also previously within their earlier life histories. It is immediately apparent that, from this perspective, the dependency conditioned upon older people in general can be aggravated or alleviated by other factors concerned with access to economic and political resources earlier in life. The impact of life course experiences associated with class, gender, race and disability on old age has to be illuminated and leads to an understanding of *differentiation* between older people in terms of their experience of, and condition, in old age. Finally, feminists have begun to weave another strand of understanding which acknowledges the importance of life history and the life-long interplay of personality and structural factors in mediating the experience of old age (Macdonald and Rich 1984; Hemmings 1985; Ford and Sinclair 1987; Hughes and Mtezuka 1992). The *subjective* meaning of life and its important constituent elements in old age have to be understood (Thompson 1992). The iconography of old age has thus changed from victim to survivor, from passive to active, from recipient to instigator, from powerless to empowered, from consumers of services to citizens with rights.

Conclusion

Theories of ageing not only offer competing perspectives for understanding the ageing process and the circumstances and experiences associated with old age, they each embody a particular view of the relative importance of individual characteristics and social factors. Each is also based on an underlying assumption about what it is to be human in general and what it is to be an old human in particular.

Notwithstanding the undeniable fact that people change as they progress from birth to death and that the biological pattern shows very broad similarities across different individuals and groups, ageing itself is not wholly or even predominantly a biological process. One only has to consider one's current position in life, be it young, middle-aged or old, to understand that biology has contributed but a very small part of the whole panorama. Furthermore, the biological and psychological perspectives on ageing, by concentrating only on very vulnerable older people, have fashioned a general stereotype of old age as a time of decline and negativity – in short, an ageist view.

The thesis adopted in this book accepts the need to locate the individual within his or her life history and current social circumstances, and to synthesize the picture of the older person as an essential component in the individual–societal (i.e. structural) dynamic. Older people, thereby, are not simply passive recipients, but also have the capacity to change themselves and their situations and to exercise their rights, provided the direction of social and economic policies and professional practices are towards empowerment.

2

The social condition of older people

Public debate about, and public policy towards, older people since the war have not been static. As the *numbers* of older people and the *proportion* of the population who are old have risen, so the views expressed by policy-makers and politicians have changed. The fact that Britain now has a sizeable proportion of its population over retirement age is regarded as an urgent matter for consideration at all levels. The circumstances in which these people live, the similarities which unite older people as a group, and the differences or sources of inequality between different older people are discussed less frequently.

Two particular ideologies have been developed and both have been used as the basis for arguments to reduce public spending on, and provision for, older people. The first is the image of a rising tide of dependent older people whose lack of productivity and increasing need for income maintenance and care have created a social problem of enormous proportions, the resource implications of which must be borne by that shrinking section of the population which is economically active (MacIntyre 1977). Government documents of the late 1970s and early 1980s reflected the consensus which was gathering around this view of old people as a burden on society (e.g. DHSS 1978). The second and more recent ideology suggests that, if there *were* any problems associated with the numbers of old people, these have disappeared and older people now enjoy an affluent and extended period of post-retirement leisure (Falkingham and Victor 1991). The well-off older person, or 'Woopie' as coined by Edwina Currie, the junior minister at the DHSS in 1988, was characterized as having secure financial circumstances, good health, pleasant and adequate material conditions, purchasing power and freedom to choose their preferred lifestyle. Moreover, this picture was thought to apply to the majority of older people:

It is simply no longer true that being a pensioner tends to mean being badly off . . . For most it is a time to look forward to with confidence. The modern pensioner has a great deal to contribute and a great deal to be envied.

(Moore 1989: 3)

The reasons behind both of these contentions and the extent to which they offer valid and accurate accounts of the social and economic experience of old age, supported by available evidence, will be examined through the course of this chapter.

However, before so doing it is important to understand that age is not unproblematic in terms of its use as a factor by which to define a distinct group in society. Old age is not a life-long characteristic like, say, gender or race. It is a state towards which individuals progress and when they reach old age they bring with them the accumulated circumstances, attributes and experience they have acquired throughout life. On the one hand, then, older people will share *commonalities* through their shared status as older people living in a society with particular attitudes, images, provision and policies towards retirement and old age. Thus, it is important to identify and document those characteristics of older people which distinguish them as a social group from the rest of the population. On the other hand, it is important to acknowledge the *diversity* which exists between older people and the extent to which other sources of inequalities, such as social class, gender or race, have shaped earlier life circumstances which are then carried into and compounded by old age. This chapter will first summarize the demographic trends and their consequences for an ageing population, then consider the factors which characterize older people as a social group and, finally, examine the sources of inequality and their impact on subgroups of the older population.

Old people in society: The demography of ageing

Population ageing

The population structure of Western European countries including Britain has changed significantly since the turn of the century. Whereas in 1901 just over 6 per cent of the population were at or over current pension age (60 years for women, 65 years for men), this figure rose steadily from about the 1920s to reach 18 per cent in 1991 (OPCS 1991). At the same time, the proportion of children under 16 fell from 35 to 20 per cent. Thus, the age structure of the population has changed from one in which young people predominated to a society in which people at the other end of the life span constitute a substantial proportion of the total population. Furthermore, projections suggest that this structure will remain stable for some time before the trend towards population ageing increases around the year 2025, when the proportion of pensioners is expected to be 22 per cent (OPCS 1991). At the same time as the elderly population has increased in relative terms, the numbers of older people in absolute terms have also risen considerably, from just over 2 million in 1901 to about 10.5 million in 1991.

While individual ageing is an inevitable and universal process, population ageing is neither. Changes in the age profile of a population are a response to social and other conditions and populations can become younger or older depending upon the impact of those conditions. The ageing of populations in developed countries is a consequence of increased fertility, decreased mortality and migration, although the effect of the latter has probably been minimal (Johnson and Falkingham 1992). Increased fertility earlier in the century has resulted in much larger cohorts of people with the potential to become old. Furthermore, the survival of greater numbers of these people past infancy, together with improvements in mortality at older age ranges, have resulted in the significant changes described above. There has been a consequent increase in life expectancy, to the extent that a person born in 1991 can expect to live 20 years longer than if he or she had been born in 1911 (Johnson and Falkingham 1992). The increases in life expectancy do not mean, of course, that the capacity of human beings to live longer has increased. Medical science has extended the potential for long life hardly at all. Life expectancy at birth is an average, based on the proportions of the population who survive to different ages, and its improvement is due almost entirely to decreases in infant mortality. Life expectancy for older people has improved much more modestly. For example, for a man aged 60, life expectancy has increased by about 6 years over the past 150 years (OPCS 1991).

The ageing older population

Within these overall population trends are hidden some distinct changes within the age structure of the older population itself. While the proportion of older people is projected to stabilize at 18 per cent before increasing to 22 per cent of the total population, the proportion of very old people (75 and over) within that group has risen consistently and is expected to rise even further by the year 2025, when the number anticipated is 2.9 million (CSO 1991). Thus, within the older population, the number of those in the age range 60–74 years will decrease relative to those over 75 years, as a consequence of falling birth rates earlier this century and the loss of life incurred during the Second World War. The older population is, then, itself ageing and this trend is not expected to diminish until after 2025. It has become common, because of this age structure within the older population, to identify the 'young old' and 'older old' as two distinct groups with broadly different life experiences and current demographic and socio-economic characteristics. Age as a differentiating factor among the older population will be discussed later in this chapter. However, it is statistics such as these which have been used to support the hypothesis that the older population is, and will increasingly become, a burden upon the rest of society, with the implicit assumption that older people are more likely to be economically dependent and need care. Falkingham (1989) has re-examined the extent to which increased numbers of older people result in an overall increase in dependency in society, and concluded that 'the degree of scaremongering over the ageing of the population in the last few years has been unfounded' (p. 230).

Bury and Holme (1991), in their study of people aged 90 and over, also demonstrated that very old age was not inevitably a time of major dependence and, indeed, there is some evidence that death, not old age *per se*, is the main event consuming health resources in later life. There is considerable debate about whether increased numbers of old and, in particular, very old people will lead to greater levels of dependency and need for care. Fries (1989) propounds the argument that periods of morbidity in later life will be compressed and therefore the periods for which people need medical care and support will decrease. However, his hypothesis is based upon a complex set of assumptions which has been challenged elsewhere (e.g. Grundy 1991).

Gender and race

Consideration of current and future population changes and their roots in events which occurred earlier this century should also alert us to the social histories which these generations of older people have experienced. All have lived through at least one world war; some have survived two. Others have entered the country as a result of immigration and other socio-economic policies. The gender and racial characteristics of the current population of older people are a product of a complex interplay between social policies, public health and its effect on mortality, catastrophic world events, socially con-structed lifestyles and individual life dramas. Nevertheless, as far as gender is concerned, these factors have not impinged upon one another in a random way, but have all served to expose men to death to a greater degree than women, with the consequent predominance of women in older populations. This trend also increases with age. Among the population over 60 years of age, 'women outnumber men by almost two to one, and with increasing age the proportion rises until more than two-thirds of those over 75 years are women' (Peace 1986: 61). As Peace goes on to observe, 'The world of the very old is therefore a woman's world . . .' (p. 61).

The predominance of women in old age is also expected to continue at least for the next 30 years or so, although the changes to the lifestyles of younger women in relation particularly to paid work, smoking and drinking may take its toll in future generations. Nevertheless, it has been estimated that 'in 2025 there will be 3.9 million men and 4.6 million women aged 65–79 and 1.1 million men and 1.8 million women aged over 80' (CSO 1991: 24, quoted in Tinker 1992: 17).

Despite the long-standing and continued predominance of women in the older population, public policy and provision have appeared in remarkably gender-neutral form and have failed to acknowledge or consider the impli-cations this fact may have for the way in which services are provided. For example, Finch and Groves (1985: 97), in their analysis of the impact of gender on social services provision to older people and their carers, concluded that: 'While social workers, along with most other people, may be gender-blind in their explicit thinking about older people they still can (and, it appears, often do) operate with implicit gender assumptions in their dealings with elderly clients.' Other studies have suggested that elderly men and male carers have greater access than women to support services and receive more help, and sooner (Hunt 1978; OPCS 1982; Charlesworth *et al.* 1984). Peace (1986: 71) conjectures that the basis for observed gender-based patterns of service provision lies in the belief that 'the hidden rules concerning role divisions do exist, even in extreme old age'.

In Britain, even less attention has been given to the racial and ethnic composition of the older population, although American policy and the academic gerontological literature have for some time included race as a core issue (e.g. Markides 1989). The age structure of minority ethnic populations in Britain is relatively young, with the consequence that within each group 'only a small percentage are above state pensionable age' (Arber and Ginn 1991: 16). Drawing on work by Haskey (1990), Ginn and Arber estimated that while approximately 19 per cent of the white population is over state pensionable age, the figure is 5 per cent for West Indians, 4 per cent for Indian, Chinese and Arab peoples, and 2 per cent for Africans and Pakistanis. Thus, although a sizeable number (93,000) of people from minority ethnic groups are older, they represent a very small population both of the total minority ethnic population *and* the total older population in Britain. These characteristics, needs and circumstances have not been adequately documented and there is a considerable dearth of information about this section of the older population.

Marital status

Partly reflecting the fact that women live longer than men, the single largest group within the older population in terms of marital status is widows. In the population aged 75 and over, 65 per cent of women are widowed, whereas 62 per cent of men – a very similar proportion – are still married (Tinker 1992).

Living situations

The mutually related factors of age, mortality, gender and marital status (and probably race, but we cannot say with certainty) combine to produce patterns of living in old age which reflect the consequences of these factors for different older people. Whether a person lives alone or with others has always been partly determined, for instance, by widowhood and disability, conditions which are much more likely to be experienced by older women. However, more recent social and attitudinal changes also appear to have been important, with an increasing trend for older people to live alone. The incidence of single-person households over state pensionable age more than doubled to 16 per cent between 1961 and 1989 (CSO 1991). This may reflect a general social trend throughout society towards smaller households, or may be at least in part a particular preference of older people to remain in their own homes as long as possible, even when partners die.

The patterns of living arrangements also vary with age. For all people aged 65 years and over, the single largest group (over half in 1985) live with a spouse or a spouse and others, just over a third live alone, about 7 per cent live with the family of an adult child and 5 per cent with siblings and others. However, for people aged 75 years and over, the likelihood of living alone is much greater (OPCS 1989).

Finally, the geographical location of older people is not evenly distributed throughout the towns, cities and rural communities of Britain. Certain areas have almost become retirement centres, with up to 35 per cent of the population over state pensionable age, while in some towns and inner cities less than 10 per cent of the population are in this age range (Warnes and Law 1984). The extent to which older people are a visible and acknowledged section of a local population may have a significant impact on the extent to which services for older people are identified as a priority. Furthermore, the *experience* of old age and therefore subjective feelings of well-being, satisfaction and security may be very different for an old person living, for example, in a densely populated inner-city environment populated predominantly by families with children and young people and possibly characterized by a high rate of movement in and out of the area, compared with a person living in a shire suburb where most people are older and the population is static.

Older people as a social group

The demographic characteristics paint an important contextual picture of the older population, but reveal little about the circumstances in which people live. However, reporting further facts about, say, income or wealth would not of themselves add very much more to our understanding, since the *significance* of particular levels of income need to be related to some kind of standard by which the meaning of those income levels within the context of society can be appreciated. For example, if it were simply reported that $x\%$ of older people live on a state pension of £30 per week, the significance of that information, in telling us something meaningful about the economic position of older people, can only be understood in relation to other facts. We might compare the figure of £30 with the national average wage, to the range of incomes going into different households throughout the population or a particular measure of the cost of living. While the divergence between individual older people has already been acknowledged, for instance between 'young old' and 'old old' people, and will be developed later in this chapter, older people are also identified as a distinct group within society, both in terms of socio-economic policy as well as social attitudes towards old people. This section will examine four dimensions along which older people are either treated or perceived differently from the rest of the population: income, housing, health and social attitudes.

Income

All of the evidence about *the levels of* income among old people has consistently demonstrated that, *compared with the rest of the population*, old people are the poor relations:

> . . . the existence of poverty and deprivation amongst a substantial proportion of elderly people has been a recurring theme of research on ageing and social conditions in all industrial societies. In Britain, elderly people have been shown to be the largest group living in poverty ever since information was collected systematically.
>
> (Walker 1981: 73)

However, as Walker goes on to note, poverty among older people has largely gone unchallenged and low incomes have been accepted as an inevitable consequence of old age. However, both the low levels of income evident among older people, as well as the high incidence of poverty, are at least in part a product of two aspects of public policy: the movement towards fixed and enforced retirement at specific chronological ages and the progressive reduction in the relative value of the state pension, upon which a high proportion of elderly people are solely dependent (Townsend 1981). Comparing the income of older people with that of the rest of the population demonstrates that older people are much more likely to live in poverty (i.e. at or below income support levels), are more likely to have low incomes (defined as income support levels plus 40 per cent) and are more likely to experience poverty or low income over a very long period of time (Walker 1990). Since the link between pensions and earnings was broken and pensions instead became indexed to prices, the relative value of the state pension compared with earnings has fallen since the mid-1980s and this trend will continue unless the policy of price indexing is changed. Given the large proportion of older people who are solely or largely dependent on the state pension for their income (an estimated 70 per cent of pensioners in 1987), these changes have further disadvantaged a large majority of older people.

Despite the enduring evidence of a low income and poverty among older people compared with the rest of the population, there is a view that older people generally are entering a golden age as far as income and material circumstances are concerned. This view has been fuelled both by the selective and inappropriate use of some specific statistics, and by the need for government to justify its policy of continuing to reduce public spending – in particular on social security, of which pensions and income support to older people is a significant part.

First, the fact that the real and absolute values of pensions have increased, together with the total absolute spending on social security for elderly people, have been cited by politicians and some academics as evidence of a significant rise in living standards for older people over recent years. However, partly because the baseline for pensioners' incomes was so low to start with, and partly because the living standards of other groups have also risen, the *relative* income position of older people as a group has not improved relative to the population as a whole (Walker 1988; Johnson and Falkingham 1992).

Second, the proportion of elderly people among those claiming income support has fallen and this change has been used to suggest a relative improvement among elderly people. However, as Johnson and Falkingham (1992) point out, the *number* of elderly claimants has, in fact, not fallen at all but remained stable. The decline in pensions as a *proportion* of all claimants has resulted from a substantial increase in families claiming benefit as the numbers of unemployed adults has risen during the 1980s. Thus, poverty among old people has not fallen. Rather, poverty has increased among families in the rest of the population.

Third, the evidence that recent economic policies have resulted in a significant improvement in the levels of income for a number of older people – the 'Woopies' – has been used to propagate the impression that these changes have benefited a majority of the older population. The small proportion of older people who are solicited as consumers of foreign holidays and leisure products present a reassuring and seductive image which is in danger of wrongly suggesting that this new affluence is the norm for most older people (Falkingham and Victor 1991).

Finally, there is evidence of age discrimination within the state income maintenance and benefit system itself, which appears to endorse the view that older people should expect to be impoverished and disabled, and should not expect the same state assistance as younger people to whom these misfortunes may befall. Evandrou and Falkingham (1989) have illustrated how entitlement to certain non-means-tested disability benefits, for example, are denied unless the claimant submits a first claim before reaching pensionable age. Thus, if an individual becomes disabled *after* reaching pensionable age, they are deemed ineligible, presumably on the basis of the assumption that pensioners must expect to become disabled, whereas younger people need and deserve special financial help. The implicit ageism within these benefits rules reinforces the view that the problems of poverty and disability are inherently part of old age and must be accepted – a view, no doubt, which many older people themselves internalize and which explains in part the low take-up by older people of those benefits for which they are eligible.

Overall, then, there is substantial and enduring evidence that, as a group, older people fare worse in terms of income than the rest of the population and possibly worse than any other single section of the population, and certainly any other age-cohort. Furthermore, while in part low income and poverty in old age is a consequence of life-long economic status as we shall discuss later, it is also a consequence of social and economic policies which, having instituted fixed retirement ages, then embody the implicit view that reduced income is one of the natural and inevitable consequences of the unproductive, retired status of old people, whose financial position is further compromised by a discriminatory benefit system.

Housing

Housing is not only a major determinant of standard of living through the material conditions – whether good or poor – it provides; it is also for some people a major asset, the single most significant source of wealth for homeowners and, possibly, a source of equity for the realization of additional income later in life. Thus both housing *conditions* and housing *tenure* are important variables in determining quality of life in old age.

Compared with the rest of the population, people aged 60 years and over occupy proportionately more of the substandard housing stock in this country (Tinker 1992). The English House Condition Survey, 1986, revealed that across all three main indicators of poor condition – lacking basic amenities, unfit or in poor repair – the vast majority of homes so classified were occupied by households whose head was aged 60 years or over (DoE 1988). For example, of the homes lacking five very basic amenities – a bath, sink, inside toilet, hand basin and hot and cold water at three points – 46 per cent were occupied by households with a head aged 75 years and over, and a further 38 per cent by a household headed by someone aged 60–74 years. The figures for unfit dwellings and those in poor repair are very similar (DoE 1988: 42). Furthermore, Henwood and Wicks (1985) have identified a trend that households which consist *only* of elderly people, regardless of tenure, are generally in poorer than average condition and more likely to suffer worse amenities, and that a significant minority of elderly people are living in inadequate or inappropriate housing conditions.

The condition of a house impinges not only on the quality of life of its occupants but also, if they are houseowners, on the extent to which the property can realize capital or income. As the evidence above suggests, where elderly people are owner-occupiers, their properties tend to be less valuable than those of younger households because they are more likely to be in poor condition. To this extent, wealth invested in housing tends to follow the patterns of income distribution. Older people as a group are less likely, despite a general rise in house ownership throughout society, to own their own homes and, when they do, the properties are likely to be worth less than those of younger age households (Johnson and Falkingham 1992). Finally, it remains the case that proportionately more elderly than younger people are dependent on rented accommodation and thus have no possibility of realizing any assets through home ownership. In particular, this generation of older people are twice as likely to live in privately rented unfurnished accommodation than the population generally, a total of 17 per cent of those aged 65 years and over (Johnson and Falkingham 1992: 67).

Health

Older people as a group appear to experience more incidents of acute and chronic illness than the general population, although they generally report their health to be good (OPCS 1990; Tinker 1992). They also consume proportionately more of both hospital and community-based health services. However, these apparently straightforward statistics emerge from a very complex interplay of different factors, including not only patterns of disease and ill-health but also the ways in which older patients are treated. On the one hand, it would not be surprising if, the longer one lives and has to negotiate environmental and other hazards, the more likely one is to succumb to an illness or disability. However, it is not clear whether illness in older people has been taken as seriously, and treated as rapidly or as thoroughly, as illness among younger people. The attitudes of some medical practitioners to illness in old age has been that of 'grin and bear it'. Thus, older people may not have always had the most efficacious investigation and treatment.

Furthermore, the health care received by older people may be adversely affected by developments in health economics and rationing practices within the health service. Health economists have attempted to produce various measures of the efficiency and value for money of medical interventions and treatments. Perhaps the most well-known is the QUALY (quality-adjusted-life-years), which claims to estimate both the *number* of extra life years which may result from a particular health procedure and the *quality* of the extra years gained. These are measures which present in apparently scientific form a judgement which is essentially a value judgement about who will benefit most from treatment and who will not. There has already been concern expressed by general practitioners that the kind of rationing which results from this approach may be used to discriminate against older people in the delivery of health care. For example, some hospitals and trusts no longer admit automatically a person aged 70 years or over with a coronary incident to intensive care, whereas younger people continue to receive immediate intensive care treatment. As the changes towards a market system in the delivery of health care result in more explicit rationing, it may be that age is increasingly being seen as a legitimate criterion by which to decide who will receive high-cost, high-tech treatment and who will not.

However, despite the overall picture of more ill-health among older people as a group, other evidence also suggests that ill-health and disability in old age are more a product of life-long inequalities (Victor 1991). The unhealthy consequences of poverty (Townsend and Davidson 1982; Blackburn 1991) which occur throughout life and accumulate in old age have been well documented, although the general view persists that age, *per se*, is the prime cause of illness and disability in older people. In fact, a high level of health, functional capacity and well-being exists among the older population and health differences tend to reflect more the gender, race and, in particular, socio-economic characteristics of individuals than of age itself. Thus, age itself is not the 'great leveller' in terms of health status and there is no moral or economic validity for the use of age as a criterion for rationing access to life-enhancing or life-saving treatments.

Social attitudes

Economic and other forms of discrimination against older people as a group can only prevail if the general attitude within society towards older people is either unconcerned or negative. The social construction of ageing within Britain embodies a number of stereotypes: the rocking-chair image; the awkward old woman; the dirty old man; the demented old man/person. Despite a superficial veneer of commitment to the veneration and celebration of old age, through the use of terms such as senior citizens, in practice older people as a group experience economic and social discrimination which is evident in the kinds of inequalities discussed in this section. This inequality compared with the rest of the population is real and measurable and is the product of ageism, which permeates all levels of society and which influences the way older people are treated within broad social policy, within social and health care practice and within more personal interactions generally. It also influences the way older people see themselves and the extent to which they feel able to demand equality and equitable treatment. In short, ageism results in a relative lack of power for older people as a group and thus is a source of social and economic oppression buttressed and validated by negative stereotypes and demeaning images. As Dick Crossman (1962) observed some 30 years ago, adequate financial arrangements are a necessary but not a sufficient condition for improving the lot of older people: 'What is needed first and foremost is a mental revolution which purges the repressed fear and shame that most of us feel with regard to old age' (p. 930).

Differentiation among older people

The particular circumstances of an individual older person will derive from a combination of two sets of factors. First, as an older person, he or she is more likely to experience poverty, poor housing and poor health as a result of the socio-economic and other processes which discriminate against older people as a group. Second, however, the socially constructed and other negative consequences of old age can be either further compounded or ameliorated by other factors which derive from sources of inequality or privilege which have developed throughout life: social class, gender, race, age and personal biography. All of these factors produce *differentiation* between older people and mean that some people, as they enter old age, will have acquired resources and had experiences throughout life which will now protect them from adverse consequences or will allow them to compensate for adversity should it befall them. Other people, however, will simply find that the struggle they have endured throughout life is significantly aggravated and deepened by the further decline in income, resources and possibly health as a result of joining the community of old people. Middle-class, professional, white men fare very much better than working-class, black women and the disparity between these groups in old age is not only wide but increasing.

Social class and socio-economic position earlier in life is the main source of inequality between older people and impinges not only on income differences in old age but also, through the impact of poverty throughout life, on housing, education and health, and on a wide range of resources, opportunities and personal circumstances. The accumulated impact of poverty and low income shows itself most starkly in the differences in the life chances of ever reaching retirement age. Men in professional occupations have an 80 per cent chance of living to age 65 years, whereas male manual workers have an 80 per cent chance of dying before reaching retirement age (Wilkin and Hughes 1986). However, the differential opportunities for contributing to occupational pensions and the trend towards private pension schemes for those who can afford them also mean that income levels *per se* in old age vary considerably and the differences between better off and poor old people are increasing, with the real prospect of the emergence of the 'two nations in old age' prophesied by Titmuss in 1955.

The *gender and race* of individual older people is also partly related to social class and socio-economic position: women and people from minority ethnic groups are over-represented in the poorest groups, both in the population generally and in the old population in particular. However, the impact of both of these characteristics is not exclusively economic, but also a consequence of social attitudes to women and minority groups.

In old age, women are more likely than men to live longer, experience a chronic disabling condition and live alone in poorer conditions (Walker 1987; Hughes and Mtezuka 1992). However, women are also more likely to have experienced a role as carer and dependent as a consequence of the social construction of womanhood and the duties it embodies. The *experience* of old age, with enforced economic dependency and, for some, physical dependency, may have very different subjective meanings and implications for women and men.

Older people from minority ethnic groups are also more disadvantaged than white older people across all the dimensions we have examined in this chapter: social class, income, health and housing (e.g. Norman 1985; Donaldson 1986; Haskey 1989). Black and Asian older people, in particular, will also carry into old age their experiences of racism and an awareness of their relative invisibility both within their minority ethnic communities and within the general population of older people. Both older women and people from minority ethnic groups, in different ways and for different reasons, may consequently have low expectations of the extent to which society will recognize and provide for their needs. As a consequence, their demands may be small and their voices unheard.

So far, this chapter has identified the structural factors which either collectivize or differentiate older people and it has been important to illuminate the various sources of inequality both between older people and the rest of society, as well as between older people with different class, gender and racial characteristics. However, in charting the sources of oppression, it is also important to avoid inadvertently validating those images of old age as predominantly negative and disempowering. The concepts of life history and biography enable the balance to be redressed and are important variables in understanding the ways in which these different structural or social factors interact with personality and interpersonal experiences throughout life to create unique responses to, and patterns within, old age for different individuals and subgroups (Johnson 1976; Gearing and Dant 1990). At one level, age itself is a key determinant of life history and experience. 'Older old' people have lived through two world wars and the most dramatic social, technological, political and economic changes of eight decades or more. 'Young old' people will have been adolescents or young adults with babies during the Second World War, the generation which began to initiate actively the changing roles of men and women (especially in employment), took part in the post-war reconstruction and witnessed more recently the dismantling of those welfare structures and values.

At the individual level, testimony from older people proclaims that if they are victims, they are not passive victims. Their views of life depend not only on economic and health circumstances, but on their own personalities, family ties, friendships and social networks, all of which, in turn, are partly a consequence of the whole-life biography of the individual person (e.g. Matthews 1979; Macdonald and Rich 1984; Hemmings 1985; Ford and Sinclair 1987; Bury and Holme 1991; Bytheway *et al.* 1990). Old people, whether 'young' or 'old', in this generation are 'survivors and their lives and their survival have inevitably involved the surmounting of personal and social challenges throughout this century' (Hughes and Mtezuka 1992: 232). Those experiences interact with structural and social variables in complex ways to produce diverse patterns of, adaptations to and satisfaction with life in old age (Thompson 1992). The concept of personal biography, then, does not negate the common experience of older people by individualizing them, but rather articulates the ways in which the minutiae of experiences throughout life is another context through which different older people interpret, negotiate and respond to old age.

3

Ageism and anti-ageist practice

What is ageism?

In Chapter 1, we examined the underlying assumptions and values of a range of biological, psychological and sociological theories of ageing and discovered that many have embodied unnecessarily negative and scientifically inaccurate images of older people. In Chapter 2, the information about various aspects of the social and economic circumstances of older people revealed that, while there is wide diversity *between* older people, *as a group* they seem to fare worse in relation to a variety of indicators compared with people in other social groups. The evidence was clear that older people experience considerable social and economic inequality compared with the rest of the population and with other subgroups within it. Thus it is legitimate to suppose that a wide variety of social policies are also based, implicitly or otherwise, on a set of assumptions or attitudes which (1) allow such inequality to be generated and (2) permit it to continue unchallenged. How is it that the diverse and disparate worlds of biological, psychological and sociological academia, medicine, incomes maintenance systems, housing systems and wider economic and social policy-making, all appear to be based upon, and to reflect at least in part, similar attitudes, values and assumptions? What are the processes by which attitudes, values and ideologies are translated into theories, policies and procedures which then influence the nature and shape of older people's lives?

The answers to these and similar questions lie in a consideration of ageism, in trying to define ageism and in understanding the processes by which it influences and mediates social experience. If we are to challenge the view, implicit in much of the public and political discourse about old age, that older people are socially redundant, we must understand better the processes by which negative attitudes towards older people are (1) generated and sustained and (2) translated into, and used to legitimate, discriminatory treatment of old people as a group along a range of social, welfare, economic and political dimensions.

Ageism is not simply another 'ism', and the nexus of ageism – old age – bears important distinctions from some of the other human characteristics which have also been identified as sources of social inequality and discrimination. Unlike race or gender, for example, old age is not a condition into which a person is born, nor is it therefore a fixed social identity. We are all ageing and old age is a condition we move towards throughout life. Thus, it is also theoretically and in principle a state which *could* be achieved by everyone and *will* be achieved by all who survive. While some people die earlier in life, old age is *potentially* a universal characteristic unlike, say, gender which is fixed. And yet old people as a group appear to be perceived as if they were a different 'minority', and old age is treated as if it were a differentiating variable, conferring a fixed social identity on those within the group and disconnecting old age from the other age-related life phases and experiences which precede it. Thus, age is *interpreted* 'as a basic source of biological variation between people and over the life course' (Bytheway and Johnson 1990: 30). The implication of this interpretation is that old people are defined as biologically, and therefore in other ways, fundamentally different from other people. This contradiction, 'it would seem, is the special characteristic of ageism' (Bytheway and Johnson 1990: 34).

The reasons why old age has been imbued in this singular way with negative attitudes and discriminatory consequences are likely to lie in a number of different arenas. First, it is important to remember that ageism is not universally evident across all cultures and societies. It appears to be especially prevalent in some Western capitalist societies, although it is increasingly being challenged in others, especially the United States. Anthropological studies have suggested that very different attitudes prevail in other societies where old age is venerated and old people ascribed high status. Thus, social attitudes to old age must develop in part in response to the historical legacy and cultural traditions of a particular society. Second, attitudes may also develop from the structure of a society, in particular its economic structure and the relationship between the economic, social and political systems. The economic redundancy enforced on older people by the policies of fixed retirement ages in most Western societies, for example, may contribute to and legitimate the view that older people are also socially and politically redundant, and therefore to be marginalized (Phillipson 1972).

Finally, the existence of old people may touch deeply atavistic fears about death and the appearance of very old people may resonate with images associated with wizards, witches and mystics. Older people present us with the prospects of our own mortality and the bodily changes associated with very long life. Ageism may also be a social response designed to protect the not-yet-old from dwelling too long on some painful, unpalatable but inalienable aspects of our futures. 'Old people' are always *other* people, never oneself, however old one may be (Thompson 1992).

Ageism, then, is a matrix of beliefs and attitudes which legitimates the use of age as a means of identifying a particular *social* group, which portrays the members of that group in negative, stereotypical terms and which consequently generates and reinforces a fear of the ageing process and a denigration of older people. The consequences of ageism are to be observed in the social and economic *policies* which discriminate against older people as a group in the allocation of resources of all kinds; in the *attitudes and values* of people generally in society and the ways these shape the treatment of, and behaviour towards, older people in both professional and personal encounters; in the *experiences* of older people and the ways in which old age, and attitudes to it, interact with other aspects of social identity such as race, gender, sexuality and disability to manufacture highly personalized experiences as well as feelings about oneself as an old person (Biggs 1993). It is for these reasons that ageism is important.

Why is ageism important: The process of discrimination

Ageism, and its constituent attitudes and beliefs, are part of a process which translates *ideas* into *experience*. It is important to understand that although ideas are not concrete objects, and therefore are sometimes difficult to consider, they do determine and shape the fabric and quality of life in powerful ways.

Figure 3.1 represents a way of conceptualizing the process by which ideas can determine to a significant degree the experiences of individuals through a

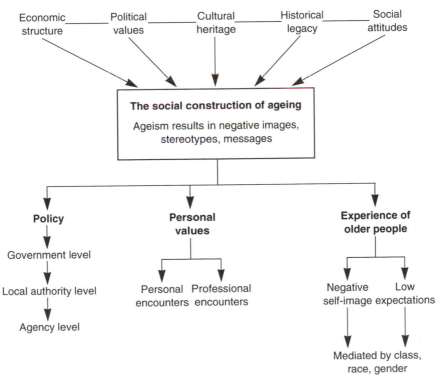

Figure 3.1   How ageism results in discrimination

number of mechanisms. As we have already discussed in Chapter 1, a *social construction of ageing* – that is, an image of old age and older people derived from the array of prevailing political, economic and social attitudes as well as cultural and social histories – becomes established and is continually reinforced by icons (in drama, advertising, literature) by powerful commentators (politicians, teachers) and through family life. This is not to argue that there exists an explicit and conscious conspiracy to propagate negative images of older people. The process is much more pervading and subtle. Rather, ideas gather momentum, become established and in so doing acquire a status of 'truth'. While some people may challenge the prevailing wisdom, on balance it prevails, especially if it is implicitly supporting other important systems such as the economic structure.

The iconography of old age as portrayed through ageism, then, seeps into people's lives via a number of routes: policy, values and experience.

Policy

Individuals and groups of people make policy and, therefore, in so far as a negative image of old age is part of the panoply of prevailing attitudes and taken-for-granted truths, the policy-makers themselves may have internalized to some degree ageist attitudes. This is evident on a number of levels. The outcomes of central government policy on income maintenance for older people have already been illustrated in Chapter 2, with some examples of explicit discrimination in relation to the exclusion of elderly disabled people from a number of disability benefits. Older people as a group experience considerable inequality as a result of a wide range of national policies. However, at the local level old people also experience discrimination. For example, many transport authorities no longer allow concessionary fares to be paid during peak hours on the grounds that older people do not have to rush to get to work and can therefore travel at cheap rates at other times. Within social services departments, the allocation of particular resources discriminates against older people. The use of trained and qualified workers tends to be much more limited in teams working with older people compared with, say, child protection. The level of training of nurses on wards for elderly people reflects a similar pattern. While untrained or less qualified staff may be able to perform satisfactorily, this allocation of its scarce trained staff to other kinds of work clearly represents agencies' views that caring for older people is easier, less demanding and less complex than that required with other groups of people.

Personal values

Ageism, like any powerful social ideology, will affect everyone in society to some degree; we are all, in part, a product of the values and attitudes around us and it is through individual people that ideas find expression in action and words. Thus, our behaviour to others will be shaped by ageist values, either because we have internalized them in part as our own, or because we have identified ageism, rejected it as a value base and are actively trying to challenge its ascendency. Personal values will have an impact on our social/familial encounters and our professional encounters with older people, and it is not always easy to recognize our own behaviour as ageist. For example, the way we address people in professional interaction should reflect an equal respect for older people as for others, whereas many professionals *assume* that old people, like children, can be addressed on first name terms. How much easier it is to be tetchy or short-tempered with someone whom one feels is, and treats as, less powerful than oneself.

Personal experience

Older people themselves are not immune from the impact of negative imagery about old age and, indeed, many old people choose not to define themselves as such (Thompson 1992). As others have reported in relation to women, some older people may have internalized a negative self-image consistent with the social stereotype. Bytheway and Johnson (1990) have cautioned against this view, lest it be taken to mean that older people may be held responsible for some of the negative experiences to which they are subjected. Nevertheless, it would be equally dangerous to ignore the impact on older people themselves of prevailing imagery, since, at the very least, this may result in low expectations among part of the older population and a diffidence about challenging the discriminatory treatment they receive. The professional must be aware of this possibility in order to be able to assist all older people as effectively as possible.

The values of an anti-ageist perspective

The values which must underpin the desire to implement an anti-ageist perspective in both personal encounters and professional practice are both simple and complex: simple in their expression but highly complex in their translation into behaviour and practice. The translation of values into principles, and principles into practice, is not straightforward. It is endemic to the process that, at each step along the way, there is no simple 'right' answer, but rather another series of questions or dilemmas to be resolved, or caveats and qualifications to be considered. The process of trying to work out how best to express in our personal behaviour and professional practice a set of anti-discriminatory values and principles is one in which there ought to be no place for the certainty of politically correct edits. It is *not* the prerogative of the younger professional to know what is right. It *is* the obligation of the younger professional to *explore* what is right – or, more realistically, what is best or the best possible – in any particular situation with an individual older person. The process therefore involves a synthesis of knowledge and values, with the professional skill and judgement to apply those attributes to a particular circumstance *with* a particular older person.

The fundamental values which provide a foundation from which principles and practice can be developed are personhood, citizenship and celebration.

Personhood

A belief in personhood perceives the older individual as a person, first, and old, second. However, this is not to be taken as a means of accepting old age by denying its existence. It is rather a value which embodies the view that this individual, her current situation and all her previous life experiences, is a valid person and of equal status and importance, through personhood, to any other individual at any age. The value of personhood ascribes to people at all ages the authenticity and worth of being alive and of having lived. The conscious articulation and application of the value of personhood to old people therefore *reconnects* old age to the rest of the life course which people travel.

Citizenship

The concept of citizenship is slightly different and concerns the relationship between the individual and society, and how that relationship is defined. There has been a trend away from citizenship towards the concept of consumer, a shift which has changed the relationship between the individual and society from one of rights and responsibilities to one defined by market relations and purchasing power. Indeed, many of the changes within the welfare system have been designed to reconstruct the user–provider relationship as one which simulates a purchasing relationship, on the assumption that she who pays the piper can call the tune. However, the role of consumer does little to empower unless the person is given the wherewithal to engage in the system of exchange. Engagement also depends not only on purchasing power, or purchasing power by proxy as enshrined in the community care arrangements, but on the ability, competence and confidence to negotiate with providers and significant others.

The development of an anti-discriminatory perspective cannot depend on the concept of the older person as consumer, since, as we have seen, older people as a group are already relatively disadvantaged socially, economically and politically. The concept of citizenship, with its emphasis on rights for the individual and reciprocal responsibilities for both the individual and society, is more relevant to an anti-ageist value base, since it postulates the validity of the older person not only as a person but also as an equally important and valid *member of society*.

Celebration

Finally, it is important that the value base celebrates old age and acknowledges that the attainment of old age is a noteworthy achievement both for the individual and, in so far as more and more people are living longer, for society as a whole. Celebration is not to be confused with the patronizing sentimentality behind such comments as 'Isn't he good for his age', nor the denial beneath the praise for an older woman who does not 'look old'. Celebration is rather the quiet validation of diversity among older people and an acceptance that old age is an authentic period of life to be valued in its own right.

The principles of anti-ageist practice

The values identified above indicate the overall direction in which personal attitudes, behaviour and practice have to proceed and provide an over-arching framework within which these details can be elaborated further. The next stage in the process of translating values into action is the articulation of a set of principles, consistent with those values and against which particular practice alternatives might be evaluated. The following principles can also be used as a set of *criteria* against which the *outcome* of a particular practice or intervention for the older person might be evaluated. How far practice achieves some of these outcomes and embodies these principles will determine how far the practice is 'good enough' in terms of implementing an anti-ageist perspective.

- *Empowerment*: the process and outcome of practice should be aimed at changing the relative power between the older person, professionals, family if necessary and other significant people to ensure that the older person continues to have, or acquires, control over his or her own life and all that goes with power and control – freedom, autonomy, dignity and feelings of personal self-worth.
- *Participation*: the meaningful sharing with, and involvement of, the older person in practice is both a key principle in its own right as well as a means of demonstrating a commitment to empowerment.
- *Choice*: the ability to make choices and to determine as far as one can the outcome of events is an important means of personal validation, as well as a right in terms of personhood and citizenship.
- *Integration*: as far as possible, people seem to want to live in mixed communities and not segregated only with people with whom they might share one particular characteristic. Celebrating old age as a valid point on the continuum of life, and not a separate, different end-phase, means integrating older people into the mainstream of life at every level.
- *Normalization*: involves making available whatever is necessary to enable old people to carry on living in the same way, with the same or better quality of life as other people in society.

Principles into practice

The specification of key values and principles is a relatively easy task; the difficulty lies in translating principles into practice. This is partly because such concepts are more amenable to discussion in the abstract than in terms of their explicit manifestation in human thought and activity. However, the difficulty is also compounded by the fact that translating anti-discriminatory principles into practice is not a one-dimensional process, with an inevitable link between value, principle and consequent professional behaviour. The particular way in which practice is executed depends more upon a process of negotiation, during which the professional and older people must, together, face a number of dilemmas and contradictory demands. Many factors intervene in this process, so that the pathway through to, for example, empowerment and choice is such that the ideal can often not be realized. Rather, the pathway for each person and his or her situation will be a product of how far the professional worker can anticipate and negotiate obstacles and problems and achieve an outcome which, in all the circumstances, is the best possible in terms of the principles of an anti-ageist approach. This is not an inherently pessimistic view; rather, it is an important stance which recognizes the complexity of the human situations to which professionals must relate and the extent to which some of the characteristics of those human situations have been created by structural factors outside of the professional sphere of influence.

Professionals who are trying to translate anti-ageist principles must accommodate within their day-to-day practice and interactions with older people a number of contradictory positions. For example:

- They must recognize the discrimination which affects *all* older people, but avoid stereotypes and acknowledge the diversity which arises from gender, race, class, life history and other factors.
- In trying to ameliorate the disadvantages and problems facing many older people with whom health and welfare professionals work, they must also acknowledge the strengths and resources which older people have acquired through life and which they bring to their old age.
- They must begin from the older person's subjective view of his or her current circumstances, but also accept responsibility for their own professional judgement, derived from knowledge and experience. Anti-ageist practice is not synonymous with always *agreeing with* the older person's point of view, although *acceptance* of his or her perspective as valid is essential.
- Professionals must try and incorporate into their practice the older person's views and yet not be limited by low expectations or the internalized acceptance by some older people of the consequences of ageism (Hughes and Mtezuka 1992).
- The older person must be seen in the context of his or her whole-life experience, but this must not be used as a reason for intruding too deeply or prematurely into personal history.
- While acknowledging the impact of ageist values and discriminatory policies on older people, professionals must avoid conceptualizing older people as victims. Their status as survivors, as people with responsibility for their own actions and with as wide a range of personalities as in other groups of people, must be acknowledged.

Thus, the detailed way in which the referral of an individual older person is managed by health and welfare professionals, and the extent to which it could be said to be anti-ageist, will depend to a significant degree on a professional's sensitivity to the practice dilemmas inherent in implementing anti-discriminatory practice and his ability to question himself and negotiate such dilemmas along the way. This requires not only commitment to anti-discriminatory practice, applied with professional expertise of various kinds, but also professional confidence. The implementation of anti-discriminatory practice involves difficult dilemmas. It also frequently involves conflict of various kinds: conflict of opinion between different professionals or between professional, older person and carer; conflict of interest between different family members, each of whom may have vested interests in different outcomes to problematic situations; internal conflict for the older person between what she may want to do and what she feels she ought to do; internal conflict for the professional between what is desirable and what is possible. The management of conflict, particularly in the context of trying to achieve such objectives as empowerment and choice, demands a considerable degree of professional confidence and the ability to accept responsibility, mediate and take decisions – actions which may, on the face of things, appear to contradict some of the principles underlying anti-discriminatory practice.

However, without professional confidence and the understanding that anti-discriminatory practice cannot be defined as a series of politically correct edicts, professionals run the risk of abdicating responsibility for helping in the complex human situations which face many older people on the basis of the misguided premise that professional judgement or decision-making is, by definition, inconsistent with an anti-discriminatory approach. Professionals must *share* their power and use it, as far as possible, to the benefit of older people and their families. However, that is very different from either giving power away or trying to deny, wrongly, that they have no power in the first place. In order to develop and challenge their own values and practice, committed anti-ageist professionals must begin by acknowledging the professional power base and finding ways of exercising authority and using professional knowledge and skills in conjunction with older people and their families.

PART II

Skills

4

Communicating with older people: The professional encounter

Introduction

For the professional working with older people, the following question arises: 'Are special skills necessary to communicate effectively with older people?' The answer must be both 'no' and 'yes'. On the one hand, it is an important stage in the development of anti-ageist practice to acknowledge that professional encounters with older people demand the same level of skill and expertise as those undertaken with other service users. Thus, older people do not need special skills: it would indeed be a step forward if, in general terms, workers and agencies demanded the same standards of interpersonal practice with older people that are regarded as essential with children, adults with mental health problems and others. However, on the other hand, the answer must also be 'yes' in so far as it is necessary to recognize that older people as a group are more likely to have experienced certain social, personal or health conditions which have a direct bearing on communication. The development of communication skills and the effective management of interpersonal encounters with older people therefore present the worker with a double agenda. First, the principles of good standards of anti-discriminatory practice in professional communication must be examined in relation to older people and the particular implications for direct work must be articulated in sufficient detail to enable practice to improve generally. Second, interwoven with this generalized approach must be the understanding of the impact of being old and of conditions more commonly associated with old age on the ability of old people and usually younger professionals to communicate effectively together. These two objectives, then, are the primary themes of the anti-ageist agenda in relation to professional encounters and communication with older people. This chapter explores the implications of these themes for practice and begins to sketch out the detail of how communication and interpersonal skills can be executed in an anti-ageist manner. The issues to be considered in professional communication are complex and interrelated. This chapter will examine the *contextual issues* which must be understood in working directly with older people; the *process of professional communication* and the skills needed to manage the process effectively; and then *the interpersonal skills* and issues which are important in communication with older people. Some specific techniques such as counselling, life review and reminiscence are critically examined in Chapter 7.

Contextual issues

The context of most professional encounters involves an older person and a professional worker who is usually younger and sometimes very much younger. This not only represents an age difference, as important as that may be in its own right. It also reflects a 'cohort difference' (Knight 1986) and marks the fact that older people and workers belong to groups whose journey through history and experience of life have been very different. While the differences between a professional and a service user are always important dimensions to be considered in all aspects of professional helping, they are particularly important when they relate to experiences which have been lived by one party but are distant history to the other. For embedded within personal and historical life events are not only the factual accounts of what took place, but also social attitudes and values, both of the wider society and of the particular microcosm of which an individual older person was a part. Current generations of older people have also lived through the global trauma of one and perhaps two world wars, the impact of which on their lives then and on their views of life now cannot easily be empathetically understood by younger generations of people (Peace 1986).

Context refers not only, however, to life contexts, but also to contemporary contextual differences between worker and service user. Here again the importance of such differences is particularly heightened in relation to older people, in the sense that they have reached a life stage yet to be achieved by the professional worker. In work with other groups of people, professionals may have experienced similar life stages or roles upon the basis of which a degree of empathy may be claimed. However, old age is a future to which they can only aspire, but of which, as a life stage, they have no personal knowledge. Furthermore, as a period of life closer inevitably to death, old age may be a part of the human condition which the younger worker is reluctant or feels emotionally less able to explore.

Context also refers to those other factors, not specifically derived from being old, which characterize the current life and previous histories of individual old people and which accentuate the differences between worker and user: class, race, gender, the history of personal relationships and experience, personality (Thompson 1992). All of these factors interact with and contribute to the experience of old age, and to personal attitudes and values, and consequently influence both the perceptions which the worker and user have of each other and their receptivity and ability to communicate.

Finally, there are contextual issues which arise from specific conditions which impair speech or understanding and which therefore have to be accommodated as far as possible in order for communication to take place. Some of these conditions are easily identifiable and their impact on communication is well known (for example, aphasia or dysphasia after a stroke, moderate or severe dementia). However, others such as depression or hearing loss are not only often overlooked in older people and their symptoms likely to be ascribed instead to 'old age', but also their impact on communication is less readily understood. The ways in which contextual issues at these different levels may be manifested and therefore influence the effectiveness of interpersonal encounters can be summarized as follows:

1 *Old people's perceptions of professionals.* The impact of previous life history and, for contemporary cohorts of working-class people in particular, of experiencing welfare provision in the context of the Poor Law, may contribute to a negative view of helping professionals and a perception of help as charity. If a particular older person is also physically dependent to some degree, these effects are likely to be aggravated as the feelings of dependency he or she brings from previous social experience is reinforced by the reality of dependency arising from current personal circumstances. The manifestation of such feelings and their impact on communication will vary and may result in passivity, withdrawal, over-compliance, excessive demands, rejection or aggression. The lack of understanding among the population generally about helping professionals and the work they do has been well documented (Mayer and Timms 1969; Sainsbury *et al.* 1982). The role of a professional worker in the mind of the older person, who has perhaps not previously had contact with welfare providers, may be coloured with some confusion or misunderstanding. For example, for many people, social services and social security are indistinguishable and both are referred to as 'the social'. The particular duties of practice nurses, health visitors, district nurses, community psychiatric nurses and domiciliary care organizers may be perfectly clear to agencies and workers (although the increased blurring of roles may tax even these agents themselves), but there is no reason why a service user should be expected to make such distinctions. And yet, the older person cannot begin to feel in control if she or he does not have as clear a view as possible of the welfare map and the positions within it of the various professionals coming to the door.

2 *Professionals' perceptions of old age.* While many agencies have begun to embrace the principles of an anti-ageist approach, it remains the case that the practice of many helpers fails to incorporate those principles into their day-to-day work and this is often manifested in their communication with older people. Professionals whose implicit values and attitudes about old age are framed in negative or unfulfilling terms cannot convey positive attitudes and values within their practice and their communication will be characterized, however unconsciously, by features which treat older people in disempowering or even demeaning ways. Furthermore, the contextual differences in life experiences may mean that the professional lacks an important knowledge base within which some of the current circumstances and behaviour of an individual older person needs to be understood. The old

person is then seen as 'only-ever-having-been-old', without the effort being made to understand previous life experiences and roles, knowledge which might also help the worker to connect with and achieve a different perspective of the older service user.

3 *The impact of ageism.* The mutual perceptions of an older person and a professional helper are in part products of cohort and age differences. However, they are also in part a result of prevailing attitudes and values to old age and a manifestation of the way global or 'macro' social attitudes feed into and influence 'micro' or interpersonal interactions between individuals. Furthermore, it is not only professionals whose perceptions are open to such influences. Older people themselves may internalize to varying degrees the prevailing social constructions, and this will colour in one way or another their views about themselves as old people. Some may reject negative stereotypes but do so in ways which deny their old age (Thompson 1992). For others, the result may be low expectations and a reluctance to make demands of the welfare system (Faragher 1978). The various ways in which negative stereotypes of women influence the socialization of girls and their subsequent behaviour as young people and adults has received considerable attention (Langan and Day 1992). The subtle and complex ways in which these processes contribute to women's self-esteem, self-identity, confidence and therefore behaviour (including communication in various different contexts) have been subject to fairly thorough examination. There has developed a body of theoretical knowledge and conceptualization which avoids portraying women as merely victims of social determinism, but at the same time acknowledges the power of the social construction of woman-hood to shape to some extent the lives of women. Discourses and images of old age influence through similar mechanisms the views older people hold of themselves and their peers and will therefore have an impact, in one way or another, on communication (Biggs 1993).

4 *Impact of other social factors.* While old age and ageism are powerful mediators of perceptions on both sides of the helping relationship, old people are people first and their age sits alongside other characteristics which, of themselves, have an important influence on interpersonal encounters. The life-long experiences of old people as shaped, in part, by class, gender, race, disability and sexuality; the perceived and actual differences along these dimensions between the helper and helped person; and the impact on self-esteem and identity, are all likely to be significant issues which need to be negotiated in the professional encounter. While the worker may share certain of these characteristics with the older person and be able initially to use any commonality as a tentative bridge to empathy, she or he must also be wary of assuming that a common characteristic is tantamount to common experience. Clearly it is not. The helper's credibility lies as much in avoiding precipitous assumptions and the drawing of false parallels between self and older person, as it does in the sensitive exploration of common experience as a basis for understanding.

5 *The impact of specific conditions.* So far we have examined the impact of a range of characteristics, attitudes and values on the self-perceptions of older people and the mutual perceptions between older people and professionals which

may arise from differences in experience and attitude. The underlying hypothesis has been that experience, perceptions, attitudes, values and expectations are fundamentally important issues to be considered and negotiated in communication between individual older people and helpers. The professional worker has an obligation to be aware of the impact of these factors and to apply that understanding to facilitate communication and endeavour to maximize its effectiveness and relevance to the older person.

However, there are also specific conditions which affect the ability to communicate through an adverse impact on physical speech, cognitive functioning or mood. The ability to speak, or speak clearly, can be impaired by a number of physical conditions such as a stroke, brain damage or illnesses which result in damage to the mouth or throat. Specific techniques must be explored in order to help the individual communicate by other means (Hull and Griffin 1989). Mental infirmity presents particular challenges to communication and, when severe, demands specialized techniques. However, general principles and skills remain applicable and, indeed, are especially important to emphasize, in order to avoid depersonalizing or infantilizing older people whose cognitive functioning results in an impaired ability to understand the world around them.

Finally, depression and hearing loss can result in withdrawal and social isolation. Both conditions frequently go unrecognized in older people, yet have adverse consequences for communication. Depression is often a feature in the early stages of dementia, when the older person is aware of lapses in memory and the occurrence of inexplicable behaviour (Froggatt 1988). Depression influences both the mood and the sense of self and thereby affects the energy, motivation and confidence for human interaction. Elderly people who are depressed need similar skills and sensitivity as younger depressed people, together with the ability to balance the validation and acknowledgement of problems and difficulties with the need to promote constructive ways of coping.

The process of professional communications

The process of interpersonal communication between older people and professional helpers is, of course, greatly influenced by the quality of interpersonal skills which the worker is able to provide and these will be discussed in the next section. However, the process is also affected by a number of issues which are particular to older people, and also by skills which are more at the level of process management than the minutiae of interpersonal interaction. By 'process', I mean here the consideration of the *course* of a particular encounter from start to finish, the factors which influence the direction which communication takes and which determine whether the process has fulfilled its purpose for both communicants. Issues of *process* cannot, of course, be separated from issues of *content* – both are inextricably linked elements of communication. However, for the purposes of analysing communication in order to discern how professional practice might be improved, it is helpful to distinguish process and content, especially in terms of the somewhat different skills and issues with which each is characterized.

Key issues in the process of communication

In addition to the contextual issues described above and in part deriving from them, professionals must take account of a number of issues which are likely to be particularly important in communication with older people: expectations; the professional agenda; the tendency towards reductionism. First, for reasons concerned with all the differences which commonly exist between worker and older person, each may come to the professional encounter with very different *expectations* about its purpose, objectives and outcome. The expectations of the older person must be explored as part of the process of communication and care must be taken to clarify, reach consensus as far as possible and to methodically re-check that expectations have not changed.

Second, because of the power differential which usually exists between worker and service user and which is particularly heightened when the service user is an older person in need of some help, it is all too easy for the process of communication to become focused upon the *professional agenda*, rather than exploring the older person's agenda. Thus, in the following extract, a general practitioner who is taking great care to explain fully the medication he is prescribing and in that sense is trying to behave in an empowering way, is so closed to alternative agendas that he fails to hear Mr Jones's concerns about his throat.

Dr:	It's probably better if we change these sleeping tablets, Mr Jones, and give you something that is not so strong but which gives you more control over when you need them.
Mr Jones:	Yes, doctor. The other ones are so big as well. It's my funny throat, you see, they won't go down properly. I don't know why.
Dr:	Well, let me explain about these new tablets. You can take either one or two. Try taking one and see how you go. You may find after a week or so you won't need one every night. There are no side-effects so they're quite safe. Try them for a week and we'll talk again.
Mr Jones:	Thank you doctor. Can I crush the tablets, because I sometimes can't swallow things easily and I get a bit flustered, you see.
Dr:	Yes, you can crush them, or just take a big gulp of milk and they will go down easily.
Mr Jones:	Well, thank you doctor.

(adapted from Open University 1982)

Mr Jones is unable to ask directly about his worries and the doctor fails to 'hear' the agenda which Mr Jones himself brought to the encounter.

Finally, professional practice in various settings with older people has been characterized by a *tendency to reductionism*; that is, a tendency to see the solutions to problems in solely practical terms, to avoid complex or painful emotional issues, to provide the minimum level of service possible and to perceive older people in a limited, superficial way rather than holistically (Rowlings 1985; Bowl 1986; Wilkins and Hughes 1986).

If the tendency to reductionism is to be avoided, this must begin in our communications with older people. The process must be such that all relevant issues are entertained as possibilities by the professional helper who must exercise skilled judgement in maintaining a sensitive balance between, on the one hand, providing opportunities for the older person to discuss areas of life or feelings which may be otherwise avoided, while on the other hand not pursuing prematurely or insensitively issues which are not relevant or which the older person is not yet willing to speak about. For example, if an older person initially refuses a particular service, is that refusal an example of self-determination or does it rather reflect lack of knowledge, low expectations, anxiety, concern about the cost implications, connotations of charity or an unwillingness to 'burden' other people (Burack-Weiss and Brennan 1991)? Using communication to help empower older people is not achieved by simply taking at face value what they say to professional helpers. The fact that practice is not so simple raises a number of problematic dilemmas for the anti-ageist worker. In principle, accepting that the older person says what she means and asks for what she wants is an important value to uphold. However, the professional must also be aware of the pressures and experiences which make it more difficult for the older person to be explicit within encounters with relatively powerful professional helpers on whose assistance they may have to depend. For example, Wilson (1993), in her study of users and carers connected to a community psychiatric service, found that older people usually expressed satisfaction when asked direct questions. Direct questions tended to elicit 'polite' or 'official' responses of satisfaction. However, the use of a technique which involved no direct questions but which evaluated satisfaction indirectly through detailed accounts of the way they coped with problems and their interactions with service providers resulted in a range of positive, neutral and negative views. Wilson identifies low expectations, lack of trust in the service provider or interviewer and differences in perceptions of care between users and providers as important factors in the tendency of older people to behave (although not necessarily think) compliantly in relation to expressions both of need and satisfaction with provision. Sensitivity to these dilemmas is essential if the tendency to reductionism in professional encounters is to be challenged.

Skills of process management

There are a number of skills which the professional worker must use during communication which are concerned more with the management of the process. They may be considered 'meta' skills – that is, they are exercised 'above' the micro skills of interpersonal engagement, although they are executed at the same time and are directed at steering the process rather than eliciting specific content. These management skills can be summarized as follows:

- planning and preparation
- beginning

- observation
- cognitive processing
- directing
- negotiating
- ending
- analysing/evaluating

Planning and preparation involve trying to predict some of the issues to be discussed as well as trying to take account of factors which may facilitate the communication: contextual issues; the personal characteristics of the older person and helper; setting; atmosphere; anticipating difficult areas. Preparation should also include consideration of issues the professional worker may find difficult.

Beginning the encounter can be an important determinant of the quality of the subsequent dialogue and needs careful planning, including introductions and explanations.

Observation is a key skill to be employed in process management, and provides information which may need to be fed back during an interview. For example, 'You looked a bit anxious just now when we talked about your son. Is there something worrying you?' Observation is also particularly important in the assessment of circumstances which may be difficult to talk about openly, such as family conflict or abuse.

Cognitive processing is one of the most important but neglected skills. It involves the processing and formulation of information *at the same time* as the interactive process is continuing. Everyone has this skill, as illustrated by the way we make snap judgements about new people based on a rapid formulation of verbal and non-verbal information received during a first meeting or even a brief introduction. The judgements may not be valid, but our mental processes immediately begin to receive information and, at the same time, assess that information in relation to the already acquired knowledge and values derived from previous experiences. The professional must harness this skill by first making explicit the process to which our brains leap instinctively. In this way, the professional not only tests and challenges the 'beginning judgements' to which cognitive processing is leading, but also, therefore, can consciously seek other information which will reinforce or counter those beginning judgements.

Directing the professional interview is the responsibility of the worker, but this does not imply overtly controlling or formal behaviour. Taking the responsibility for the direction of an encounter means trying to ensure that all relevant areas are explored and that the encounter satisfies as far as possible the objectives of the older person, the worker and, if appropriate, the carer or family.

Negotiation will often be a part of the management of the process, especially if the interview is to meet the needs and objectives of all parties. The worker may need to negotiate discussion of issues which are important but sensitive or difficult. He or she may also need to negotiate between the older person and carer that specific items, of importance to one party or the other, are included.

Ending an encounter in an appropriate and clear way is very important, although the detail of how the ending takes place will depend upon the content, purpose and level of emotion contained within the interview. Drawing an encounter to a close, and leaving the older person and/or family with a clear view of both what has been achieved and what is to follow, including tasks agreed, are key skills in process management.

Analysis and evaluation should also be regarded as part of the management of interactive processes, since it is these skills which (1) attempt to 'make sense' of what occurred and the information exchanged and (2) link any individual interview with those preceding and following it. Analysing and evaluating are cognitive skills of assessment which can be undertaken by the worker alone, in supervision or in conjunction with the older person/family, as appropriate.

Interpersonal skills

The skills involved in communicating with older people are essentially those required for good professional communication with adults generally, with the important proviso that they must be applied within the context of an understanding of the experience of ageing and the impact of ageism. At the level of interpersonal interaction, this implies at the outset a power differential between worker and older person which may interfere with communication, and therefore particular account needs to be taken of it. The skills employed in any one encounter will also vary according to:

- *Purpose*: is the interview mainly for information-giving in relation to a particular task or is it exploratory or directed at counselling?
- *Scope*: is this a one-off interview or part of a series of contacts?
- *Content*: are the issues likely to be highly charged emotionally or concerned more with day-to-day matters?
- *Abilities*: does the older person experience any impediments to communication (psychological, physical, mental)? How able or experienced is the worker in applying any special skills required?

Verbal skills

Verbal skills are one of the main media of interpersonal communication and various elements are important for professional helpers to incorporate into their practice:

Listening. Paradoxically, refraining from speech during periods of listening is a core skill (Scrutton 1989). However, the listening must be *active* by which is meant that the worker must be consciously *hearing* what is being said, *demonstrating non-verbally* that they are listening, *observing* the manner and particular emotions which accompany the speech, and *cognitively processing* all this information. Many professionals do not listen actively, are not able to tolerate the silences that can prompt user speech and are not skilled in facilitating the older person's active participation (Lishman 1994).

Facilitation. This involves the worker in either trying to change the direction of an interview, exploring other areas of discussion or enabling the older person to begin to address more difficult issues. The most important skill is the ability to ask questions in ways which are open rather than closed. Many professionals ask closed questions which either require only a 'yes' or 'no' answer or, which in their formulation, presume a particular response. For example, Mrs Vernon is 81 years old, has run her catering business and been active in local politics and voluntary groups. Her husband, Joe, disabled for many years, has recently died. They had been married 52 years. Compare the following two extracts:

Extract 1

Mrs Vernon: It's funny being here on my own after all these years together.

Worker: You must be very upset now Joe's died.

Mrs Vernon: Well, yes, I supose so. But I'll cope. I'll always cope. Always will, somehow.

Extract 2

Mrs Vernon: It's funny being here on my own after all these years together.

Worker: How did you feel when Joe died?

Mrs Vernon: Well, I miss him, of course I really do miss him but I was also relieved, I have to say. I nursed him all those years and seeing him in so much pain and, at the end, it was a relief. That sounds awful doesn't it?

Worker: Many people feel like that, especially after looking after someone they love for so long. How will you feel on your own?

The first extract, with the worker presuming a particular response, elicited only avoidance, expressed as superficial clichés, from Mrs Vernon. The second example, with an open-ended question about feelings, enabled Mrs Vernon to articulate a much more complex set of feelings about her husband's death and her current circumstances.

Responding. The worker must also respond to the service user in ways which sustain and develop the communication. Responding skills include clarification, summarizing, reflecting back, acknowledgement and confirmation. These skills are executed verbally but are often accompanied by reinforcing non-verbal gestures, such as leaning forwards or backwards, hand movements, eye contact and so on.

Verbal speech must be clear and the words used should be appropriate and not full of technical language or jargon. This is not because of an assumption that older people cannot understand such terms, but rather because the insensitive use of technical or professionally specific language carries with it the covert message that the worker is more powerful. Use of language is important and extends also to terms of address: it is an abuse of professional position to make assumptions about how to address a service user. First names should not be used without permission or invitation.

With older people whose ability to speak, or speak clearly, is impaired, special skills must be applied. These might include techniques such as writing, gesticulating or a shared code of bodily movements. The inability to hear speech is also an impairment which adversely affects communication and often goes unrecognized, and is seen as an inevitable part of ageing or as an indication of declining mental abilities (Hull 1989). Awareness of the possibility of hearing loss, which may have a gradual onset, ought to be part of the knowledge the professional worker brings to their communication with older people. If suspected or confirmed, the worker can employ some fairly simple techniques to maximize hearing potential and minimize the adverse impact of hearing loss on communication: reducing background noise; engaging eye contact securely; facing the person directly and talking clearly without other non-verbal distractions; ensuring the face is visible; adjusting the pace and pitch of speech but not shouting; checking for understanding periodically and asking straightforwardly if certain issues need repeating or explaining. In cases of severe or total hearing loss, the professional and older person may need an interpreter, although the worker must take care to talk *to* the older person and maintain full eye contact and engagement with him or her.

Non-verbal skills

The non-verbal accompaniments to speech constitute another set of core communication skills, whose importance is not sufficiently recognized:

Observation. These skills are crucial, particularly in providing clues or information about feelings and meanings rather than the factual content of spoken words. It is through observation that the worker may be alerted to trends which should be followed, emotional issues beneath the surface or anxieties which it is difficult to express. Careful observation is also important to assess well-being or otherwise, and most non-medical professionals are ill-equipped with knowledge about the appearance of older bodies. While many might be able to recognize the physical signs of a health problem from the appearance and behaviour of a young child, few can do so in relation to old people. How does older skin bruise, for example? What is the significance of cloudy eyes? Is it 'normal' for an older person to sit in a chair all day?

Appearance. The older person is also able to observe and therefore the professional's appearance – and the messages it sends to the older person – is an important dimension of which workers should be aware. Appearance and demeanour should suggest a balance between approachability and professional competence and should convey respect for the older people to whom the professional is offering a service.

Body language. The stance and gestures which accompany verbal communication send independent messages to the service user. It is important that body language both conveys the messages intended and that these non-verbal communications are reinforcements rather than contradictions of what is being said. Body language is also a powerful medium for the creation of positive atmospheres, to help people relax and to convey warmth. Insensitivity about body language can, conversely, result in negative effects and impede communication.

Facial language. Maintaining eye contact and using facial gestures such as smiling to engage are both important, but facial expressions generally are often the least controlled of communication media. A look can pass across the face without the wearer having any time to prevent it, but it will be observed and understood by the receiver.

Touch. The use of physical touch merits special attention. Older people who have lost partners or lived alone for many years may be acutely deprived of physical touch and welcome a hand or arm at appropriate times. However, because older people tend to be seen as less powerful than adults generally and may be infantilized by professional helpers as a consequence, an over-readiness to touch may show an expression of unconscious discrimination. This is an issue which requires careful and sensitive judgement, and such factors as gender, class or cultural differences between the older person and the professional may be important.

Exploration

It is important to state that exploration, not only of facts but of feelings and meanings, should be a feature of communication with older people. The evidence suggests that professional communication is often limited to that necessary for finding a practical solution to a specified practical problem (Rowlings 1985). Thus, the emotional, social and developmental aspects of older people's lives have often been ignored. Again, the use of exploratory techniques requires sensitivity and judgement, and should not be applied unnecessarily or prematurely. However, providing the *opportunity* for exploring areas of life other than those central to the practical problems of daily living is a recognition of our acceptance that older people are not one-dimensional, but have inner lives and interpersonal relationships like other people.

Handling emotional issues

There are two sets of skills which are important here. First, the ability to *recognize* when an emotional problem might be present and, second, to be able to *work constructively with expressions of emotion* and emotional problems when they arise. Recognition of the possibility of emotional issues begins with the recognition that the older person is an emotional human being. The skills of working with emotional issues demand the ability of the worker to be able to 'hold' emotions, to provide a safe arena for their expression, not to deny painful feelings, to acknowledge emotions while also enabling the older person to cope constructively with negative experiences or feelings.

Challenging

It is not inconsistent with an anti-ageist approach to recognize that communication with older people will sometimes involve challenge. The principles of empowerment and choice should not be used as an excuse to abdicate professional responsibility for introducing issues which the older person may experience as difficult. In finding solutions to life problems, older people may need to be challenged about their view of themselves, about alternative understandings of the problems they face or about their views of other key people, especially partners or family (Scrutton 1989). It is important to distinguish between confrontation or challenge as an essential element in communication, and behaviour which is confrontational. The method by which professional confrontation is executed should not be confrontational. It can be quite gentle in its delivery but still be effective as a technique for enabling an older person to reappraise. It can be difficult for younger workers to challenge older service users, not least because of the age difference and the cultural ideal of respecting elders. Ageism, with its stereotype of older, dependent, passive people, contributes also to a feeling that older people must not be 'upset' but left peacefully as far as possible in their rocking-chairs. However, while challenge is difficult, to avoid it on these grounds further depersonalizes the older person.

5

Assessment

Introduction: Assessment, needs, resources

The National Health Service and Community Care Act (1990) assigned to local authorities the lead responsibility for the coordination and production of community care assessments of individual older people and imposed a duty upon authorities to undertake a comprehensive multidisciplinary assessment for any person for whom such an assessment was deemed necessary. The Introduction to the book identified the pivotal position of comprehensive assessments within the matrix of community care arrangements. At the level of the individual service user, the comprehensive assessment is the mechanism which drives the funding and resource systems, as well as the vehicle for the implementation of key principles such as user/carer participation and choice. At the macro level of community care planning, the summation of individual comprehensive assessments and the collation of data about need, both alleviated and unmet, are key elements in the forward planning process and are catalysts to the development of new services designed to meet better and more adequately the needs of the population in a particular locality.

The legacy of professional practice

Assessment has always been a cornerstone of social work, social service and health care practice. The importance of assessment or diagnosis as the first key stage in a process which leads to intervention designed to meet need and improve a person's situation or functioning has long been recognized within professional training and practice across all aspects of social and health care. However, there is evidence that the standard of practice of assessment of older people has been, at the least, variable and has generally fallen short of the standards routinely expected and achieved in relation to other groups of people (e.g. children). Rowlings (1985) reported considerable differences in scope and content between the assessments of social workers on the one hand, and those of domiciliary care organizers and occupational therapists on the other. However, she also found wide variation in practice between different workers in the same professional group. While some responded with a restricted focus on resource-eligibility, others undertook a more expansive assessment not limited to particular service options. In general, however, research has suggested that the assessment of older people has tended to be restricted to the assessment of need for specific services, often requested by a carer, a general practitioner or other third party, and is frequently undertaken by relatively untrained ancillary staff, particularly in social services departments (Means 1981; Black *et al.* 1983; Bowl 1986). There has also been criticism of the quality of medical and paramedical assessment of older people and the tendency for some health practitioners to view medical problems as inevitable consequences of old age and therefore not as legitimate need. Part of the problem has been the absence of a foundation of professional consensus about what constitutes good assessment practice with older people. High levels of expertise and models of good practice undoubtedly exist but have remained localized and undisseminated. There has been no impetus at the local, regional or national levels to develop the kinds of models of multidisciplinary comprehensive assessment which have characterized developments in working with children and families (DoH 1991b).

The relative lack of progress in developing and disseminating models of good assessment practice with older people must be seen in part as a further reflection of their relatively low status within the professional and organizational cultures of health and welfare agencies. This, in turn, can be traced to those ageist values within society generally, which permeate social and political thinking and which thereby influence the extent to which older people as a group are viewed as less important, less in need or just less interesting than other groups of people.

The development of improved assessment practice, based upon anti-discriminatory principles, is therefore presented with a number of particular difficulties:

- a relative dearth of needs-led comprehensive assessment models upon which to draw;
- few established models of interdisciplinary collaboration and decision-making in relation to older people;
- the relatively low position of older people within the status hierarchies of medical and social service agencies;
- the lack of professional consensus and theoretical knowledge about development in old age and the consequent lack of clarity about what constitutes a good quality of life for older people (Hughes 1990);
- a reluctance to apply the concept of risk to older people and consequent low levels of ability to identify and assess risk in general and abuse in particular.

Evidence of these difficulties emerged in the four localities selected by the Social Services Inspectorate to undertake pilot projects to develop a system of multidisciplinary assessment of older people (DoH 1989b). The multidisciplinary panels established to undertake the development work experienced considerable difficulties and none was able to produce an assessment schedule which fully satisfied community care requirements, particularly in relation to comprehensiveness, user/carer participation and a needs-led approach.

A new era in assessment practice?

Taken at face value, the imperatives of the community care legislation require a considerable shift from the legacy of the past, in which assessments with older people have been limited, resource-led and lacking the foundation which comes from multidisciplinary collaboration about relevant theoretical knowledge and ways in which shared practice can be improved. Guidance on the implementation of assessment arrangements decreed, first, that where a full assessment is necessary, it should be comprehensive and needs-led, assessing the applicant's circumstances 'in the round' (DoH 1991a: 5), and 'should not focus only on the user's suitability for a particular existing scheme' (p. 18). Second, it is 'the local authority's responsibility to ensure that *all* needs are considered' (p. 9), including housing, health, financial, employment, education and other needs and that, therefore, the assessments should be multidisciplinary (p. 9). Finally, the principle of user and carer participation in the assessment process is a major theme which recurs throughout the legislation and guidance. The extent to which these three features of needs-led approach, multidisciplinary collaboration and user/carer participation can be incorporated into community care assessments depends upon a number of factors.

A key question is how we define need, a concept which is not absolute, but which depends on a number of relativities or comparisons, some of which are politically defined at the national or local level. The concept of need also has an objective component (need defined in relation to a specific standard, such as minimum income) and a subjective component, which presumably is relevant when trying to incorporate a user's view into the assessment process. Thus, the concept of need is complex and its effective application to the assessment of older people really requires the development of a much clearer consensus of what it is like to be old, what development in old age is about, and a much more affirmative view of old people. It is only in relation to such a body of knowledge and expectations that the situations of individual older people can be assessed in a positive, enhancing way. The imperative to develop a needs-led approach may be the impetus needed to engage in the difficult process of establishing such a body of knowledge and consensus. However, there are indications that this opportunity may be jeopardized by subsequent official caution that 'assessment must remain rooted in an appreciation of the realities of service provision' and that there must exist a 'high level of understanding and respect between assessors and service providers' (DoH 1991a: 14). There also now seems to be a lack of clarity about how the separation of identification of need (assessment) from the determination of service response (implementing and managing care) can be achieved. While a separation of these two stages is envisaged, other government advice advocates that the assessor and care manager should be one and the same practitioner. The dilemmas raised by the attempt to produce an assessment of need uncontaminated by an awareness of limits of resource availability, particularly if the assessor then becomes the care manager, are issues to which we will turn in Chapter 9. Here we will examine assessment as a professional activity, in terms of the process, underlying principles and different levels of assessment; we will consider the principles of anti-discriminatory assessment; a framework for conceptualizing and implementing comprehensive assessments with older people and carers will be proposed; a case example will be used to illustrate some of the practice issues which arise; and, finally, some of the dilemmas of anti-discriminatory assessment practice will be discussed.

What is assessment?

Assessment is fundamentally important to health and welfare practice, since it forms the basis of intervention and also provides the criteria upon which the effectiveness of intervention can be evaluated. Indeed, the outcome for service users depends crucially upon the quality of assessment, since intervention or service responses will only be as good as the assessments from which they emerge. Poor, limited, superficial assessments result in partial, inadequate or unsuitable responses to users and carers. Expansive, comprehensive assessments rooted firmly in professional knowledge and experience are a better foundation for a more effective meeting of need and, if services are not available, for the identification and monitoring of unmet need. This latter point is crucial. If the community care machinery is to achieve its aim of developing a wider array of more diverse services, the identification of unmet needs is a vital catalyst without which such development may not occur, even though the identification of needs which cannot be met raises difficult issues for the practitioner–user/carer relationship.

The process of assessment

It is important at the outset to recognize that, while assessment results in the production of an opinion or written statement, it is fundamentally a process; furthermore, it is a *dynamic* process and the *way* in which it is executed and the *elements* which are included have a significant impact on the quality and accuracy of the outcome. Assessment involves much more than the collection of information and data. The process incorporates a number of key components and involves the assessors (including users and carers) bringing to bear a wide range of observational, communication, interpersonal, cognitive and analytic skills: 'Assessment is about *understanding*. This entails listening, observing and relating to both what is being said and to the feeling with which this information is given' (Neill 1989: 8). Neill's analysis also points to the fact that the process of assessment involves *relationships*, primarily between practitioner, user and carer, but also different orders of relationship between different professionals or members of the wider family or community.

The aims of professional assessment are to:

- identify, clarify and define problems;
- understand the meaning or significance of problems for user and others;
- understand the meaning or significance of problems in relation to relevant prevailing knowledge and theory;
- form an opinion or alternative possible opinions (or hypotheses), which, to a greater or lesser extent, offer a systematic account or explanation of the information about a user and his or her situation;
- make recommendations about intervention (objectives, action and methods of work);
- identify resources to secure objectives;
- provide the criteria for subsequent evaluation of the intervention and reassessment.

Figure 5.1 represents diagrammatically how the process of assessment may

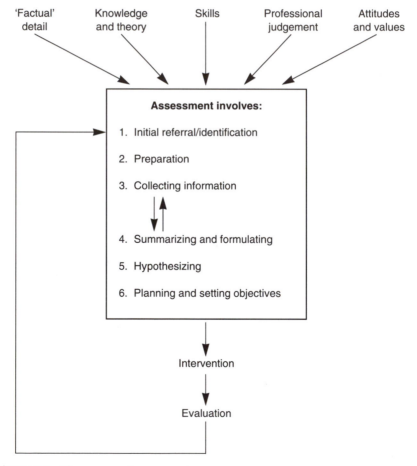

Figure 5.1   The process of assessment

be conceptualized and illustrates the fundamental importance of assessment as a basis for subsequent practice. The top of the figure identifies the various ingredients which are synthesized within the assessment process:

1 *'Factual' detail*. Information is collected during the assessment process, but it is important to recognize two issues which influence the 'factual' picture that emerges. First, factual information varies according to its quality or its 'hardness'. There is little debate about 'hard' data or information – it can be examined and affirmed and is not subjective. For example, one's level of income or a confirmed diagnosis are fairly 'hard' data. However, other 'factual' detail is often little more than opinion, however informed or professional that opinion may be. Thus views about whether a particular level of income is adequate or what impact on quality of life a particular illness will have may be given firmly but are nevertheless open to question, particularly if they are the views of other people, not the user or carer. Thus the assessing practitioner has to *discriminate* between the quality of the different sources of factual information which are presented. Second, however, the information presented will in large part be due to the lines of enquiry and investigation which the assessor initiates. Thus, if no questions are asked about a specific issue, it is less likely that information will be volunteered. This point is more than a statement of the obvious. It identifies the need for the assessor to question herself throughout the process about lines of enquiry not yet explored; to challenge an emerging view by explicitly seeking information from other sources; by constantly checking against the tendency to form an opinion too early.

2 *Knowledge and theory*. The information about any individual person or situation cannot, of itself, be useful. It can only 'make sense' if it is set against some prevailing body of knowledge or theory about similar people or similar situations, as we noted in Chapter 1. Thus, information about older people has to be assessed in relation to knowledge and theory about physiological, psychological and social ageing; gender; race; class; the impact of poverty; loss and grief; development in old age; mental health; and numerous other aspects of knowledge and theory which may be relevant in any one case.

3 *Skills*. The practitioner will need to employ a wide range of interpersonal, observational, communication, negotiation, analytic and writing skills in order to gather information and formulate meaningful understandings, or hypotheses, upon the basis of which objectives and work plans can be identified.

4 *Professional judgement*. Assessment has, on occasions, been portrayed as a technical process in which the collection of information leads inevitably to a particular conclusion. However, because the process is complex and because, in human situations, there is often no inevitable link between certain 'facts' and specific conclusions, the exercising of professional judgement and experience becomes an important ingredient. This is particularly true when the process embodies the principle of user and carer participation, a principle which could easily be translated into 'agreeing at all times with the views of the user or carer'. In the light of the low expectations of many older people, this would be a dangerous tendency and would not

lead to much improvement for many service users. Professional judgement, therefore, is a valid component of the assessment process, albeit one which must be applied flexibly and with suitable self-examination by the practitioners of the bases from which that judgement is being drawn.

5 *Attitudes and values.* Inevitably, the attitudes and values of the assessing practitioner cannot be excluded from the process and therefore their presence must be acknowledged and, as with professional judgement, their influence on the assessment process must be subjected to self-examination and criticism. Anti-discriminatory values should be paramount, but even so the practitioner's response to a particular older person can be coloured by all kinds of triggers and minutiae from past experiences, and therefore the practitioner has a professional duty to also scrutinize his or her attitudes, particularly those which arise spontaneously on first impressions.

The assessment process itself involves several elements, from the initial referral or identification through to the setting of objectives. However, these stages are not necessarily sequential: collecting information continues at the same time as the practitioner is cognitively processing that information and beginning to formulate explanations, understandings or working hypotheses. It is all too easy for the final opinion or assessment to be the product of a self-fulfilling prophecy, a process whereby an earlier opinion has been confirmed only because it has not been tested by the explicit seeking of new information or the consideration of alternatives. The prime duty of the professional is constantly to question the assessment which is emerging and, as far as possible, to subject this opinion to further testing and evidence.

The principles of anti-discriminatory assessment

Training and development work with professionals in several agencies has identified a number of essential core principles of anti-discriminatory assessment which cluster around three different levels of practice: direct practice with users/carers; interprofessional or multidisciplinary practice; management practice (Hughes 1993).

At the level of practice of individual practitioners and teams assessing older people and their carers, six core principles have been identified. The process and procedure for assessment must:

- begin from the user's and the carer's definitions of the relevant problems or issues;
- be comprehensive – that is, be flexible and adaptable to enable a wide range of factors and information to be collated, appropriate to each individual person and their circumstances;
- provide a coherent framework for understanding and prioritizing the complex information gathered from a range of different sources;
- take account of issues of confidentiality;
- offer a consistent standard of good practice to users and to carers, while also recognizing that the process of assessment involves the exercising of judgement, whether professional judgement or the subjective judgement of users and carers;

- incorporate an understanding of inequality derived through age, gender, race, class, disability and sexuality.

Second, the assessment process must embody certain principles which enable effective interprofessional dialogue and collaboration to take place. Two such essential principles are that the assessment process:

- must provide the mechanism for direct involvement and communication between different professionals at different levels in a range of different statutory, voluntary and other agencies;
- must allow for the possibility that different professionals will bring different perspectives which may result in different conclusions or recommendations as to what is a desirable outcome of the assessment process, and therefore must provide a mechanism by which such differences can be identified, recorded and, if possible, reduced.

Finally, practitioners have identified the need for management practices in their own agencies to be based on three key principles, which should ensure that management:

- provides clear guidelines, instructions and a sound framework for the comprehensive assessment process and these should be developed with practitioners;
- provides clear commitments and policy objectives both for the development of comprehensive, multidisciplinary assessments and for the kinds and levels of services which the outcome of such assessments will require;
- recognizes that comprehensive assessment should be part of a planned and structured approach to the development of services for older and disabled people, which should be based upon the principles of anti-discriminatory practice.

Different levels of assessment

While the process and principles of assessment discussed above are generally applicable to all forms of assessment, clearly there will be variations in the extent to which the process can be validly contained to a simple and brief activity or where it needs to be expanded to encompass a complex, multi-need or high-risk situation. The Social Services Inspectorate has identified a typology of six levels of assessment ranging from 'simple' to 'comprehensive' and advocates:

> . . . moving away from separate assessment procedures for different services to an integrated system that offers a graded response according to the type and level of need. This requires a specifically defined process for allocating the appropriate form of assessment.
>
> In setting up this process, managers will have to identify the type and number of assessment personnel available and their comparative levels of expertise. These can then be related to the level of demand for different

types of assessment and criteria can be developed for the allocation of assessments to different personnel.

(DoH 1991c: 43)

While this guidance envisages that assessment staff will henceforth cease to be linked to specific service provision, the implementation of this typology may, in fact, result in old arrangements for assessment continuing under another guise. For example, instead of domiciliary care organizers assessing a person for home help care, he or she will be given 'limited' assessments (i.e. those which someone has already decided need only the provision of home care). It is the point at which the decision about the appropriate level of assessment is taken, and by whom, which is crucial. The danger is, of course, that an individual user may be assigned a level of assessment which is not sufficiently comprehensive or extended, nor conducted by a practitioner with sufficient training to identify all of their needs or to assess risk appropriately. There is also the question of whether the implementation of a typology of levels of assessment involves some early decisions about the kinds and levels of resources required (in order to decide on the level of assessment) and thus whether the process effectively becomes resource-led not needs-led.

Although it is neither necessary nor appropriate for every assessment to be comprehensive, multidisciplinary and extended, it does seem necessary that, apart from specific requests for specific services where service eligibility criteria can be applied, all assessments at the outset should be considered as possibly leading to a full multidisciplinary procedure. Thus, all staff undertaking assessments should have sufficient training to enable them to identify when a more comprehensive assessment is required.

Comprehensive multidisciplinary assessment

The process of assessment, its underlying principles and the inherent issues for practitioners are, then, generic to all levels of needs-led assessment. Comprehensive assessments differ only in the scale and complexity of the assessment and therefore in the range and level of knowledge, skills and experience demanded of the practitioner. Nevertheless, the differences between, say, a situation in which the problems are clear and the risks low, and one which is characterized by high risk and unpredictability, are not just quantitative but qualitative too. That is to say, comprehensive assessments not only demand *more* knowledge and skill, they also demand different levels of knowledge and skill and, in particular, the ability to manage complexity and to integrate within the assessment process a large number of different factors and, usually, different people.

A framework for comprehensive assessment

The process of assessment, then, is complex and demands a high level of professional expertise. When the process is also comprehensive and multidisciplinary and has the objective of enabling the user and carer to participate in a meaningful, empowering way, the levels of complexity and expertise increase further. It is clear that practitioners need a framework to help them manage this process, to produce a degree of consistency of purpose, scope and content of assessment across different practitioners, while also enabling the assessment process to be adapted flexibly to individual people and their circumstances. The framework introduced here does not, of itself, provide a schedule or checklist to be completed, but rather offers a model for practice based upon the principles and definition of comprehensive multidisciplinary assessment discussed earlier and which utilizes the concepts of *quality of life* and *risk*.

The concept of the quality of life of older people, particularly in residential settings but also in the community, has been the subject of considerable research and academic interest (e.g. Hughes 1990) and has also been developed considerably for application in inspection and quality assurance procedures (e.g. DoH 1989c; Sinclair and Gibb 1990). The concept of risk has been recognized as being important in so far as older people have been defined as dependent or vulnerable (Stevenson 1989), but there has been little systematic analysis of risk, risk tolerance and risk management in relation to older people (for a discussion of these issues, see Norman 1979). However, together the two concepts offer a starting point for the development of an approach to assessment which is systematic, holistic and incorporates the principle of user and carer participation. From this starting point, the *purpose* of multidisciplinary assessment becomes the assessment of quality of life and risk. The *scope* of assessment will vary between individuals and be dependent upon the range of factors impinging upon the quality of life and the nature or level of risk faced by a particular user and carer. The *content* of the assessment should integrate the user and carer perspectives at all stages of the process, and not simply add on their views at the end. It is important, also, that user and carer definitions of what factors contribute to the quality of their lives and levels of risk are incorporated into the process.

The factors or aspects of life which determine quality of life and risk will vary between individuals. However, various sources indicate that for most people the following factors are relevant (DoH 1991d; Hughes 1993):

1 *Personal characteristics*: appearance, cultural issues, gender, race, life history, critical life events, age, expectations, satisfaction, etc.
2 *Attitude to self*: self-esteem, satisfaction with autonomy and decision-making, perceptions of constraints to one's independence, control, etc.
3 *Health*: perceptions of health, current physical and mental health, history of illness, medication, access to health resources, etc.
4 *Functioning*: ability to undertake tasks of daily living, ability to undertake personal care and care of others, etc.
5 *Environment*: both household (e.g. satisfaction with house, personal space, warmth, comfort, adaption to personal needs/abilities, resource) and locality (e.g. access to services and shops, security, location, safety, proximity to friends and family).
6 *Financial and material circumstances*: income, wealth, transport, material resources, expenditure, etc.
7 *Recreation and activities*: leisure activities, activities inside and outside the home, contacts with organization, attitudes, satisfaction, constraints on purposeful recreational activity, etc.

A. Personal dimension: The older person

	Professional view: Need/risk	Professional view: Strength/resources	User perspective	Carer perspective
1 The person				
2 Attitude to self				
3 Health				
4 Functioning				
5 Environment				
6 Finance and resources				
7 Recreation/activities				

B. Family dimension

8 Family composition and contacts				

C. Community network dimension

9 Community relationships				
10 Support network				

Figure 5.2 The assessment model: Data collection

8 *Family*: the family network, location of family members, level of contact, quality of relationships, etc.
9 *Community relationships*: significant relationships, opportunity for emotional expression, physical contact, social contacts, sexual relationships, etc.
10 *Support network*: extensive/limited nature of support network, stability of network, who provides assistance, support, etc.

These factors encompass the concepts of quality of life and risk. However, of themselves, they offer no more than a functional approach to assessment, and therefore must be organized into a framework which is based on the anti-discriminatory principles which affirm the older person (Key 1989). Thus, the framework should:

- Regard the older person – and carer if appropriate – as being at the centre of a network of personal, familial and social dimensions, which together determine his or her quality of life and level of risk.
- Provide a mechanism for identifying the perspectives and views of the user and carer, and other professionals, on each of these dimensions.
- Incorporate an approach which examines each dimension not only in terms of deficits (i.e. needs and risks), but also in terms of the strengths and resources which enhance quality of life and reduce risk, or which potentially can be mobilized to do so.

Figure 5.2 depicts this data-collection phase of the framework, and presents schematically a model which incorporates the principles identified. This method of presentation is not intended to suggest a data-collection form, with boxes to be filled in. Rather, it is a graphic representation of the various elements, dimensions and perspectives which need to be incorporated into the framework and the process of data collection.

The scope and content of the assessment defined by this framework is necessarily variable. Not all areas will be examined in the same degree of detail for every individual. However, the diversity of the range of information and its potentially extensive scope do require consideration of the *methods* by which the data may be collected and thereby offers an opportunity for the development of more creative ways of defining and discussing with older people these various areas of their lives.

First, the imperative to examine not only disabilities, needs and risks but also abilities, strengths and resources may, of itself, create an important climate of empowerment which will influence the manner in which assessment is conducted and the methods used to collect information, particularly from older people themselves. Second, the emphasis on user and carer perspectives on each dimension may lead to more participatory methods than the question-and-answer interview, which symbolizes the professional's relative power and authority. For example, constructing *with* the older person a network diagram to record information about family and support networks is a simple way of involving the user, often used with other client groups but not so much with older people (Fig. 5.3).

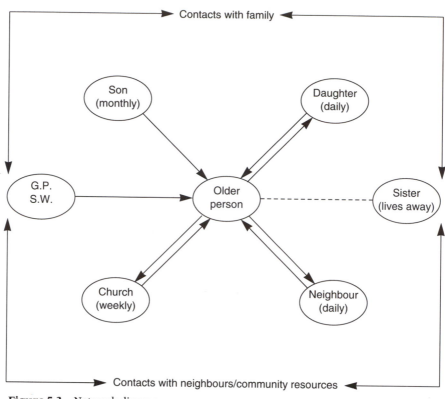

Figure 5.3   Network diagram

Similarly, the drawing with the older person of a family tree to collect information about family composition and contacts has several advantages over the
more traditional methods of information gathering. It not only involves the
user more demonstrably in the process and provides him or her with a visible
record of the interview, but also begins to construct a historical picture of the
older person. This is often an essential first step in identifying the strengths and
personal resources which an older person has developed during their lifetime.

A particularly suitable method of undertaking a comprehensive assessment
is the biographical approach and the biographically based interview method,
such as that developed in the Gloucester Care for Elderly People at Home
Project (Boulton *et al.* 1989). While a biographical approach has been
employed as a research method in a small number of studies of older people,
this was the first known systematic attempt to develop the biographical
approach as a form of health and social care *practice* aimed at assessing health
and social services needs (Gearing and Coleman, in press). Care coordinators
on the project received training in the flexible use of a biographical approach to
interviewing and assessment. It was found to produce qualitatively better
assessment and to be particularly useful in: eliciting older people's attitudes;
understanding family relationships and older person–carer relationships;

understanding why certain services may be regarded as acceptable or unacceptable; relating to older people labelled as difficult or those with dementia; understanding the impact of past life on current circumstances and future aspirations; helping with past or present traumatic events.

The process of assessment, however, is not complete until the data collected have been *summarized* and *formulated*. These essential stages in the process involve the translation of the information into understanding, and the translation of understanding into objectives and plans for action. It is at these stages of the process that the professional judgement and experience of the assessor, and her or his ability to exercise a range of analytic and negotiating skills, is of fundamental importance. The information collected will be diverse and complex, and the assessor must come to a view as to the relative importance of different pieces of information and prioritize the information into a manageable, but valid, summary. The summary must also locate the information within a context of relevant knowledge and theory. In addition, the assessor may well be faced with competing perspectives from users, carers and other professionals, with whom she or he must negotiate, liaise and consult.

These processes involve cognitive as well as interactive skills, and therefore the exercising of professional expertise and judgement cannot be eradicated from the process, as we have already noted. Rather, it should be acknowledged and, in so doing, be open to scrutiny and accountability. Nevertheless, the processes of summarizing and formulation are complex, and therefore initially it may be helpful to consider the information in relation to the three dimensions – personal, family and community – around which the data were collected. Figure 5.4 presents a graphic representation of the process of summarizing, in which the most significant information is identified and prioritized in relation to each of the three dimensions.

Furthermore, the purpose of assessment, defined earlier as the assessment of quality of life and risk, offers a means of helping the assessment to identify a focus for managing this stage of the process, when a wide range of complex information from a variety of different sources has to be summarized. The purpose of the assessment can be translated into two key questions, which provide such a focus: Overall, what is the quality of this person's life? Overall, what is the level and nature of risk she or he faces?

Finally, the formulation stage involves using the results of the assessment process to identify objectives, plans and strategies. This stage draws considerably upon the knowledge, skills and judgement of the practitioner and, as with the summary stage, may be facilitated by formulating the objectives around two key questions: How can quality of life be maximized? How can the level and nature of risk be minimized?

However, it is important that the answers to these questions remain framed in terms of needs and not in terms of specific service options at this stage. For example, if maximization of level of life and minimization of level of risk for a particular individual can best be achieved by meeting the following needs:

- adjusting to the loss of a partner
- assistance with daily tasks
- opportunities for purposeful activity

	Need/risk	Strength/resources	User perspective	Carer perspective
A. The personal dimension				
B. Family dimension				
C. Community network dimension				

Figure 5.4 Summary

it is important that these are not immediately translated by the assessor into:

- one-to-one counselling
- home help
- day centre.

These are only possible options and may not be the most appropriate or creative responses, nor might they allow for user choice. Indeed, if assessment is to lead to a coherent and integrated package of care, including both practical and therapeutic services where appropriate, it is very important that assessors express the assessment in terms of needs and resist the temptation to suggest particular resources (Humphries 1992).

CASE EXAMPLE

This case study is designed not to produce a definitive assessment, which is not possible as a paper exercise, but rather to demonstrate some aspects of the process in practice as well as issues which may arise for the practitioner.

A. Referral

Mr and Mrs Austin, aged 84 and 86 years respectively, are referred to the social services department (SSD) by the community nurse, who has been attending Mrs Austin weekly for about a year because of her dementia, incontinence and inability to care for herself. The community nurse expresses her concerns to the GP that she has heard Mr Austin shouting abusively at Mrs Austin and has seen what she believes may be finger bruising on Mrs Austin's upper arms. The GP telephones the SSD and expresses the view that Mrs Austin may now need to be in residential care.

Self-preparation

- How do you picture Mr and Mrs Austin in your mind?
- Are they black or white? Frail or fit?
- What images do you have of these two people?
- How are these images influencing your expectations?
- How might you as a younger/white/black/male/female practitioner be perceived by the Austins and how might such perceptions influence the interaction?

Self-preparation

It is important to get in touch with the attitudes, expectations and values which a referral may trigger for both the practitioner and service users.

Action

- How would you explain your visit to the Austins?
- How would you arrange the visit? By letter?
- What factors need to be considered in suggesting the time of a home visit?
- What plans would you make for the interview?
- What areas of information would you aim to cover in this initial contact?

Plans

It is important to plan specifically *how* the meeting will be arranged, *what* its purpose and objectives are and *who* will be involved.

B. Initial visit

The practitioner visits Mr and Mrs Austin at home and finds the following circumstances:

1 They live in a terraced house in an old block of houses, only two of which are still inhabited. The property is situated in a large industrial estate, surrounded by factories. There are no other houses or shops within 2 miles.

2 The inside of the house shows some signs of recent neglect and the smell is evidence of Mrs Austin's incontinence, as you later discover. However, the house is comfortable, and with small rooms and gas fires is reasonably warm. They occupy only the ground floor.

3 Next door, in the only other occupied house, lives a long-standing neighbour, a widow Mrs Booth. Both the Austins and Mrs Booth have lived in their respective houses for almost 30 years. Mrs Booth, who is 70 years old, comes into the Austin house daily and takes all the laundry, including frequent changes of bedlinen caused by Mrs Austin's incontinence.

4 Mrs Booth is at the house when you visit. She is extremely worried about her friends and says she has seen Mr Austin push his wife in a moment of frustration. She is an active person, and appears to do all the shopping for the Austins, as well as their laundry. She appears to welcome the visit with some relief.

5 Mrs Austin is fairly confused – she is unable to sustain a meaningful conversation, either lapsing into silence or into irrelevant speech. She also appears to be quite frail, unable to walk unaided from one room to another. She no longer performs any of the household tasks, but can wash herself (hands and face) and dresses herself with some assistance. You see the bruising to which the community nurse referred.

6 Mr Austin is a reasonably fit man, who has taken over both the household tasks and the physical care of his wife. He does not welcome your visit and does not cooperate willingly with any of the questions. Therefore, some areas of information such as income and his own views on their current circumstances cannot be covered. He refuses all offers of assistance and spontaneously volunteers the emphatic view that neither he nor his wife

will move to residential care. He denies he has any problems and says he does not know how the bruising occurred.

7 The Austins have a daily visit from the community nurse who bathes and toilets Mrs Austin. They have no other visitors, have no children or surviving relatives nearby.

Questions

- What are the dilemmas involved in ascertaining the *wishes* of all three parties, in view of Mrs Austin's mental condition?
- Overall, what is the quality of life for these people and can it be improved?
- Overall, what are the risks inherent in the current situation and can these be reduced?

C. Initial assessment

The practitioner completes an initial summary of the information obtained so far, and argues the case for moving towards a comprehensive assessment.

Initial assessment: Mr and Mrs Austin

Initial referral. Mr and Mrs Austin were referred to this department by the community nurse in August this year. The causes of concern at this stage were:

(i) evidence of bruising to Mrs Austin's arms, with the suggestion of current and previous physical abuse of Mrs Austin, possibly by her husband;

(ii) Mrs Austin's confused mental state and the level of care she requires;

(iii) Mr Austin's ability to care for his wife and himself in their own home.

This initial assessment is based upon one visit to the Austins, discussion with Mrs Booth (a neighbour) and telephone conversations with CN and GP.

Mrs Austin is an 86-year-old white woman. Physically, she appears to be well – her skin is a good colour, her eyes are bright, she appears to be reasonably well nourished, although fairly thin and quite frail.

In terms of functional abilities, she can walk on flat terrain only with assistance, but not stairs. Her gait consists of small steps and shuffles and I would anticipate she may not be able to walk far or negotiate uneven ground very well. She can wash her face and hands; she can dress herself but needs help to put clothes on in the correct order. She is incontinent of urine and occasionally of faeces if not toiletted regularly, done day and night.

Mentally, she appears to have little short-term memory but will speak of events long ago. She appears to recognize her husband as her carer, but it is unclear whether she understands her relationship to him. Her speech is often very repetitive. She responds to instructions and requests and appears to understand what is said some of the time. However, on the day of my visit, she was very withdrawn.

Mr Austin informed me she occasionally resists help but is not directly violent to him or Mrs Booth. Mr Austin has tranquillizing medication from the

GP to give if and when necessary. He says he uses this only at night, when otherwise Mrs Austin is often up and about, in order that he can sleep.

Mr Austin is an 84-year-old white man. He appears to be physically well and able to perform the normal range of household tasks, although somewhat slowly from my observation.

Mentally, he is alert with good short-term and longer-term memory. He appeared to be tired and drawn, however, and was impatient at times during the interview. He may be depressed; his mood was flat and he seemed anxious. He is also fairly thin, although he tells me he cooks and that he and his wife are well fed.

Mrs Booth is a neighbour who visits daily. Seen only briefly: appeared lively, mobile, active and in good health and mood.

Relationship. It is extremely difficult to assess the quality of the current and past relationship between Mr and Mrs Austin in the present circumstances. Whatever the past relationship, Mrs Austin is unable now to provide the emotional support and intellectual stimulation which a mentally able partner could provide. Mr Austin is facing the prospect of watching his wife's ability to recognize and relate to him, and to their past life together, gradually disappear.

Mr Austin emphatically denies hurting Mrs A. However, the evidence suggests he may have done so, and Mrs Booth confirms this.

Details of their past relationship are not yet available.

Networks

1 The Austins are extremely isolated and very vulnerable. Their network consists of:

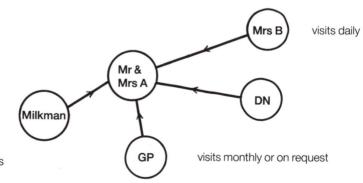

The Austins rarely go out. Mr Austin goes for a walk occasionally or to shop when Mrs Booth sits in the house. Mrs Booth does most of their shopping.

2 The Austins and Mrs Booth together comprise a system which, at the most, maintains a degree of equilibrium, although at some cost to all three members. However, the equilibrium is precarious in that only a small change in any one element of the system could cause its collapse. The risk of collapse is therefore very high.

Material conditions. The downstairs of the house is warm with cooking and heating facilities. General conditions in the house are comfortable but neglected. The kitchen, particularly, shows signs of neglect and needs to be properly cleaned.

The accommodation in use consists of kitchen, living room, downstairs bedroom, outside toilet. Upstairs – only the bathroom is used. The other upstairs rooms are furnished but have not been used for a year or so.

Financial circumstances. These are unknown and Mr Austin was unwilling to discuss. They will receive state pension but may or may not be receiving supplementary income support or an occupational pension. (Mr Austin worked as a storekeeper in a large retail firm.)

Summary and formulation. The main causes of concern are:

1 The risk of physical abuse to Mrs Austin
2 Mrs Austin's mental condition and its effect on her and Mr Austin
3 The vulnerability and social isolation of the Austins
4 The vulnerability of the current support system
5 The deteriorating material (and financial?) circumstances.

Hypotheses (the 'why'). There are a number of alternative hypotheses:

1 The change in Mrs Austin's mental abilities has created both physical and emotional stress for Mr Austin as primary carer, resulting in depression (very common among older people) and uncharacteristic stress-related behaviour (hitting his wife). If so, the provision of practical and emotional support (or other alternatives) will reduce the risks to both Mr and Mrs Austin.
2 The continued viability of the current system is in question and the risk of breakdown is high. While Mr Austin is primarily responsible for care, Mrs Booth is pivotal and, as a woman, appears to undertake most of the domestic tasks.
3 The physical abuse may reflect a long-standing pattern of behaviour within the marriage compounded, but not caused, by the stress of current circumstances. The pattern of domestic violence may be associated with alcohol or drug misuse. In this case, the risk of continued abuse may continue even if stress is alleviated through support.

Recommendation. To undertake a comprehensive assessment.

D. The comprehensive assessment

Objectives

1 To establish relationships and try and engage the three people, but particularly Mr Austin, in the process.
2 To gather a wide range of information about past and current circumstances as well as attitudes and feelings about the future.

3 To obtain a specialist assessment of Mrs Austin's mental state, its causes and prognosis.
4 To observe Mr and Mrs Austin together.
5 To identify needs/risks of all three people in the system.
6 To identify the strengths/resources of all three people.
7 To draw conclusions about overall quality of life and risk.
8 To explore further the three hypotheses identified at initial assessment.

Who will be involved?

1 Mr and Mrs Austin and Mrs Booth: How can the practitioner balance the need to assess each person individually but also as a couple and a system?
2 GP and community nurse: How will their views about residential care be evaluated? What issues does this raise for the consultation process?
3 Consultant psychogeriatrician: Why has Mrs Austin not been referred before? What issues would the request for such a referral raise for Mr Austin? For the GP?
4 Other sources: Housing department? Voluntary organizations? Disabled living advisor? Occupational therapist?

What knowledge/theory may the practitioner need? For example:

The ageing process	Risk assessment
Dementia	Crisis intervention
Depression	Task-centred work
Alcohol/drug abuse	
Recognition of elder abuse	Life biography
Grief and loss	Attachment
	Life course
Social networks	Self-identity and -esteem
Gender and caring	Interpersonal relationships
Domestic violence	Marital relationships
Systems theory	
Inequality/poverty	

What skills may the practitioner have to draw upon? For example:

Counselling	Observation
Engaging an unwilling person	Communication
Negotiation	
Liaison	Thinking
Consultation	Prioritizing
	Summarizing
Management	Analysing
Organization	Evaluating
Administration	Reasoning

What values should underpin the process? For example:

- In terms of *user choice*, who is the user in this situation? How can different choices of different people be accommodated?
- In terms of *user participation*, how can all three people participate appropriately? How can Mrs Austin's interests and views be represented?
- In terms of *anti-ageist practice*, how can the process validate and affirm the current strengths of the people concerned as well as past achievements, while also acknowledging need and risk?
- How can these values be communicated to the service users and demonstrated in the way the assessment process is executed?

E. 'Making sense': Developing alternative hypotheses

Whatever the comprehensive assessment concludes about the levels of need/risk and potential or actual strengths/resources, at initial assessment the practitioner identified three alternative hypotheses, or three alternative ways of understanding some of the information which was available at that time. It is important that the assessment investigates further the validity of each of these alternatives, since each one may have different implications for the decisions about the best possible package of service options. The three alternative hypotheses identified could be described as:

1 Carer Strain Theory
2 System Breakdown Theory
3 Domestic Violence Theory

The process from formulation of hypothesis to the determination of service outcome is represented in Table 5.1.

In order to demonstrate clearly the process of analysis, the hypotheses have been presented so far as alternatives. However, in a real situation, they are not necessarily mutually exclusive. For example, Mr Austin may be under additional strain as carer and have a history of domestic violence. Nevertheless, it is important to identify the dominant, or most likely, hypothesis in order to draw conclusions on the priorities of need and service options.

Dilemmas in anti-discriminatory assessment practice

Practitioners should not underestimate the shift in practice required to implement a needs-led approach to assessment of older people. A commitment ideologically and professionally to a holistic assessment of need and risk, rather than the assessment of eligibility for service, is a necessary but not a sufficient condition for effective assessment practice. New skills, as well as attitudes, have to be developed. Key (1989) portrays the essential shift as one from functional assessment of abilities and selective assessment of criteria for rationed services to one of 'affirmative assessment' through 'a unique individual profile, from which an individualised plan for the person is developed through a more equal relationship with the elder being assessed' (p. 69).

The practitioner is responsible for bringing to the process a wide range of

Table 5.1 Developing alternative hypotheses

Carer Strain Theory	System Stress Theory	Domestic Violence Theory
The demands of Mrs Austin's condition fall mainly on Mr Austin, causing increased emotional and physical strain.	The system involving the Austins and Mrs Booth is in a precarious equilibrium with much strain falling on Mrs Booth, without whom the current system may collapse.	The physical abuse is a long-standing feature of the marital relationship.
This results in impaired coping with the demands of day-to-day living and increased tension.	The current system and the respective roles of Mr Austin and Mrs Booth has probably evolved in response to a deteriorating situation and may not represent the wishes of either to carry on caring to the same degree.	The situation (both in terms of risk of abuse and ability to care) is aggravated but not primarily due to Mrs Austin's mental frailty.
This is heightened by the particular nature of Mrs Austin's mental frailty and her consequent failure to relate to her husband who is also grieving for the loss of the relationship.	To avoid breakdown, the current system may need to be either strengthened by support, or replaced in part. The position of Mrs Booth is pivotal and her wishes need to be clarified. The current situation appears to be one of incipient crisis.	Mrs Austin can no longer care for herself and no longer protect herself. The opportunities and triggers for abuse will increase, as will the demands of caring. Mrs Austin is vulnerable and her protection is a key issue.
Standards of living fall: social isolation increases; physical abuse may occur. Poor quality of life and high risk develop.	The adequacy of current standards of living is precarious; crisis results in tension, leading to frustration and abuse. The various interests of the three people in the system are in conflict to some degree.	A situation of crisis, tension and vulnerability is the dominant picture.
Primary needs are: (i) emotional support for carer, (ii) practical support for carer, (iii) maximizing Mrs Austin's residual abilities.	Primary needs are: (i) a stronger support system, (ii) maximizing the quality of life of all three people, (iii) minimizing the risk of system breakdown.	Primary needs are: (i) to protect Mrs Austin, (ii) to improve her residual abilities where possible, (iii) to improve the quality of life.

Table 5.1 continued

Carer Strain Theory	System Stress Theory	Domestic Violence Theory
Appropriate services could be: (i) counselling/group support for Mr Austin, (ii) support service package, (iii) rehabilitation/group activity for Mrs Austin.	Appropriate services could be: (i) task-centred approach to identifying common goals, (ii) strengthening or replacing elements of the current system with support services.	Appropriate services could be: (i) intensive home support to both monitor and provide care, (ii) professional intervention with Mr Austin to address the abuse, (iii) preparation of options to remove Mrs Austin if necessary.

knowledge and theoretical perspectives about the kinds of needs and risks which older people may face, and the ways in which these are mediated by gender, race, class, life history and circumstances of a person's life. The application of this knowledge involves sensitive judgement and skill. A needs-led approach should begin from, but not be restricted to, the user's definition, as this may be limited by low expectations or lack of knowledge about resources (Fisher 1991). The practitioner must be able to analyse the interconnectedness of needs and identify underlying causes, beginning with the service user and carer, but also moving the focus beyond what may be their limited horizons. This requires a sensitive, exploratory approach which validates the user/carer perspective but integrates with it the knowledge and skills of the practitioner. The thesis propounded by Hughes and Mtezuka (1992: 236) in their analysis of social work and older women is relevant to all older people:

> Most importantly, the assessment must be conducted *with* the older woman. It must incorporate her views of her situation and her needs and yet not be limited by her low expectations and internalised acceptance of the consequences of ageism and sexism.

However, the role of the practitioner *vis-à-vis* the user/carer may not be easy to marry with the role of the practitioner as an employee of an agency responsible for the provision, either directly or indirectly, of services which will be rationed. This raises two possible dilemmas which the practitioner will have to manage. First, in relation to users and carers, the practitioner may well be aware that she is identifying and discussing needs which are unlikely to be met within the current limits and range of available services. It is important that individual assessments do identify such needs, since it is precisely this information, collated over time, which is meant to inform the overall process of forward planning by agencies. However, this dilemma creates a potential tension in the user/carer–practitioner relationship and it may be professionally difficult for the practitioner to contemplate raising expectations which are unlikely to be met. Second, the role poses a corresponding potential tension in the practitioner's relationship with the employing agency:

> The needs-led approach alters the nature of the practitioner's account-ability to the employing agency and to the user . . . under new arrange-ments, practitioners will be expected to sustain with integrity a measure of independence from both parties, while safeguarding the interests of both.
>
> (DoH 1991c: 111)

This in turn implies increased autonomy for practitioners involved in assessment.

A related issue, but one which deserves its own consideration, is the centrality of user/carer participation and the way in which the assessment process can be used to empower users and carers. Practitioners need a clear understanding of the processes by which social inequalities of various forms are derived from prejudicial and stereotypical attitudes. The development of this understanding and its translation into anti-discriminatory practice has been a subject of discussion for some time in relation to gender, race and, more recently, disability. However, as we have noted throughout this book, an understanding of ageism, its impact on the lives of older people and its interaction with sexism and racism is much less advanced. The incorporation of an anti-ageist approach to practice is important not only to the definitions of quality and life and risk in older age, but also to the development of anti-discriminatory ways of communicating with, assessing and working with older people (Hughes 1990; Hughes and Mtezuka 1992). As with all attempts to develop an anti-discriminatory approach, the process raises dilemmas for the practitioner:

> Some of the inherent tensions and contradictions of anti-discriminatory practice are brought into especially sharp relief during the assessment process. For example, a commitment to acknowledging and validating personal biography must not be a justification for intruding too deeply or too early into a woman's personal history. The commitment to assessing needs in a gender-sensitive as opposed to gender-biased way must not be a reason for ignoring the way old women define their roles. The legitimate aim of raising the consciousness and expectations of old women must not be used to deny old women the right to determine their own future and lifestyles.
>
> (Hughes and Mtezuka 1992: 237)

These principles apply to work with all older people. The participation of users and carers – a desired outcome of empowerment – will require the practitioner to be highly skilled in facilitation, negotiation, representation and advocacy. Meaningful participation also implies that the user and carer are well-informed (Fisher 1991). Effective participation involves the creation of a climate which is open and safe and within which differences of opinion, painful emotions, deep-seated fears, anxieties or aspirations can be explored. It is arguably the practitioner's responsibility for creating such a climate.

Finally, the achievement of a needs-led approach, multidisciplinary working and user/carer participation is dependent significantly upon the interpersonal and management skills of the practitioner. Interpersonal skills are crucial, since it is largely through the medium of interpersonal communication that the assessment process is conducted. As the coordinator of a process involving a wide range of different individuals and agencies, the practitioner must be able to communicate effectively with people from very different backgrounds and with different perspectives, attitudes and levels of expertise. I have already referred to the range of skills needed to facilitate the effective participation of the user and carer. In relation to professionals and other relevant individuals, the practitioner will need to be able to assimilate the different professional perspectives, negotiate around those perspectives if necessary, and coordinate the communications received from a variety of sources. These interpersonal skills are closely connected to the necessary management skills, especially when the assessing practitioner meets conflicting opinions, conflict of interest or simply conflict between individuals. In these instances, the practitioner must be able to address conflict, if possible reduce it and, if not, come to a professional judgement as to how conflict can be managed. Management also refers to the skills required to orchestrate the assessment process itself, from initiation, liaison, coordination, formulation and conclusion.

In conclusion, it is clear that, as Michael Key (1989:66) has noted, '. . . improving the practice of assessing elders is one of the challenges facing practitioners'. The National Health Service and Community Care Act (1990) offers the possibility, but by no means the certainty, that assessment practice will be improved and developed into the comprehensive needs- and risk-led approach which is essential to improving the quality of life of older people.

6

Implementing and managing care

Introduction

The Introduction to this book described the evolution of the concept of care management which has appeared in most official literature in Britain and noted the process by which the concept of 'case management' was transmuted into 'care management'. In America and Canada, *case management* was essentially designed as a response to service fragmentation, poor coordination and low levels of service options (Moxley 1989). Its objectives were the improved integration of services and the individualization of need, as well as the development of a more diverse range and increased levels of service provision. The importance of 'evaluation and exploration' within a case management approach was implicit and derived from the tradition of using the 'case' as the focus of both service delivery and evaluation in clinical and client-led models of service provision (Huxley 1993).

The largely unnoticed and unquestioned slippage to the term 'care management' in Britain is more than a semantic tidying-up, argues Huxley (1993): it represents the adoption of a terminology which has no 'empirical referents' (p. 367) and, therefore, can be used to mean a number of different things to different people. There is evidence of confusion about precisely what care management is and how it can best be operationalized in practice (Fisher 1991). A mass of literature has emerged to try and explain the various models and the organizational arrangements designed for their implementation (Renshaw *et al.* 1988; Allen 1990; Beardshaw and Towell 1990; DoH 1991c, 1991d). Furthermore, whatever care management as a system of service provision and delivery might mean, its implementation has also been used as the vehicle for a political agenda of introducing market principles and structures into the organization and delivery of welfare. Thus, care management has been linked inextricably to the so-called 'purchaser–provider split' in much of the literature, despite the fact that such a link is neither essential nor, arguably, desirable (Cambridge 1992).

The implications of the articulation of a care management approach with an internal market structure and consumeristic principles will be examined in more detail later. However, in the light of the confusion about care management, it is important to clarify what this chapter is about and to explain the terminology which has been used. In the light of the variety of ways in which community care arrangements have been implemented in different agencies, particularly in respect of whether 'assessment' and 'care management' are undertaken by the same person, this chapter will not use the term 'care management'. Here we examine specific elements of the care management process; namely, those concerned with the implementation of the care plan agreed at assessment and the management of the package of services provided. I will, however, use the term 'care manager' to refer to the person who undertakes these roles and tasks and the reader must bear in mind that this may or may not be the same individual who has been responsible for orchestrating the comprehensive assessment.

The role of the care manager

There has been considerable debate as to whether the care manager role is new and certainly it demands many of the skills traditionally associated with most of the professionals involved in care provision in the social services, health and voluntary sectors (Orme and Glastonbury 1993). However, there is also evidence that older people as a group have not hitherto been afforded the professional skills of needs-led assessment and systematic coordination of services. Older people have tended to receive a one-off response, usually from an existing service, as a means of containing a crisis.

How, then, does the care manager role differ from the roles with which health and social services practitioners are already familiar? The precise answer to this question depends crucially upon whether the care manager is responsible to some degree for a budget and resource allocation or whether the role is limited to one of coordination of services whose extensiveness and level of provision is decided by a more senior manager. Each of these models has different strengths and weaknesses, as well as implications for the skills and tasks required of the care manager. These will be discussed later, but first it is worth noting the similarities and differences between the care manager role and other practitioner roles in helping agencies. Øvretreit (1993) has identified a hierarchy of roles which overlap and require the execution of many similar skills, but each of which also involves a different balance between management and profession-specific tasks:

- *Caseworker*: the practitioner has responsibility for a case (an individual person or family network) and is primarily responsible for providing specialist professional services (e.g. home nursing, family therapy, support, medication).
- *Keyworker*: the practitioner as the named worker for an individual or family, usually employed by the agency identified as providing the most relevant

services for a particular case. Implicit in the role is the need to liaise with other professionals and informal carers and the responsibility of the keyworker is to provide a human link between the service user and a range of services.

- *Case coordinator*: the coordination role is explicit in this example, and usually means that there has also been an agreement about the need for several practitioners and agencies to be involved. The case coordinator usually provides some services directly as part of the care package.
- *Care manager*: under the new arrangements, the care manager will have either indirect knowledge of, or direct responsibility for, the budget within which care must be provided. In addition, the care manager, at least in theory, has some authority to implement and monitor a range of services, including those provided by agencies other than her own employer. In practice, however, the ability to mobilize and ensure the quality of such services will depend crucially upon the care manager's skills of negotiation and ability to manage conflict or professional difference. The care manager may or may not provide services directly to the user.

All four of these roles may involve both direct *service provision* (support, interpersonal or medical therapy, counselling, profession-specific services) and the *management of networks* (individuals in the family, professionals, agencies). However, the balance between these two elements is different. For the caseworker, the emphasis will be on direct professional service provision, although clearly that will require liaison with other people, management, at least, of the individual family network, and possibly the coordination of less significant inputs from other service providers. The keyworker role explicitly emphasizes liaison and shifts the balance slightly towards management, while this shift is taken even further with the case coordinator role. However, the care manager role is at a point along the direct service provision–management spectrum which, in practice, could involve very little, if any, direct professional service provision at all from the care manager.

Two approaches to the care manager role

The extent to which the care manager has direct or indirect responsibility for a budget or resource allocation between the competing needs of different service users is a crucial factor in determining the nature of the role. Beardshaw and Towell (1990) have noted the emergence of two different models around which the various diverse trends within implementation have crystallized: the social entrepreneurship approach and the service brokerage approach.

Social entrepreneurship describes the model developed within the projects designed and evaluated by the Personal Social Services Research Unit (PSSRU) at the University of Kent (Challis and Davies 1986; Challis 1987; Challis *et al.* 1990). The essential feature of this approach is the delegation to the care manager either of the predetermined budget for a single case (at single worker level) or of the predetermined budget for a locality (at team manager level). Theoretically, the responsibility for budget and resource allocation is the catalyst for the development of new and more flexible services which match better the needs of the service user and it is this model which relies most heavily on a consumerist approach as a basic rationale. In practice, however, the model embodies an inherent tension between the implementation of a needs-led assessment in the context of both a limited budget and the task of deciding on the relative priorities of the needs of different service users and families. Arguably, the relationship between care manager and service user will inevitably be coloured by these conflicting responsibilities: how far will the care manager's responsibility for implementing a care package to meet need be compromised by the responsibility to the agency for budget management? The extent to which the care manager can be an effective advocate may be challenged.

Service brokerage describes an approach in which advocacy with and on behalf of the service user is to the fore. In this model, the care manager's key role is to broker and bargain for the best package of services to meet an individual's defined and agreed needs. Unencumbered by resource allocation responsibilities, the emphasis is upon the protection of individual rights, quality assurance and evaluation. Even within this model, there may be tension between the advocacy role and the brokerage role: the latter may involve compromises with service providers, which conflict with the service objectives for which the care manager has been advocating. However, one of the main weaknesses of this approach is the lack of leverage or power which the care manager has with service providers, not only to obtain services but to demand different and more relevant kinds of services (Dant and Gearing 1990). This weakness is particularly heightened if the care manager is completely independent of the main service-providing agencies, for example a worker in a voluntary agency or a care manager appointed by the service user.

Essential tasks in managing care

Whichever model or combination of models is adopted in a particular agency, the care manager will undertake a number of key tasks essential to the process of implementation and subsequent maintenance, monitoring and review of care packages. The Department of Health (1991d) has identified eleven key tasks:

- determine user/care participation
- agree pace of implementation
- confirm budget
- check service availability
- renegotiate existing services
- contract with new services
- test options
- revise care plans and costings
- establish monitoring arrangements
- monitor
- review

However, if the carer manager's role is to include not only the achievement of 'the stated objectives of the care plan with the minimum intervention necessary' (p. 71) but also the empowerment of user/carer and maximization of choice, this

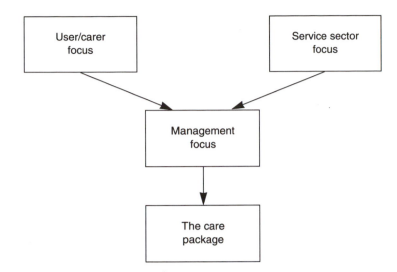

Figure 6.1   The care manager role

list omits some crucial tasks. A more comprehensive breakdown of the elements within the care manager's role suggests a range of tasks focused on (1) the user/carer, (2) the service sectors and (3) the management function.

The *user/carer focus* includes establishing agreements, agreeing pace and timing, agreeing priorities and checking satisfaction. The *service sector focus* includes brokering for services, contracting for services, agreeing specifications, agreeing service levels, defining arrangements for delivery of service and developing new services. The *management function* includes resource allocation, budget management, securing choice, recording the details, establishing monitoring arrangements, monitoring the arrangements, evaluating the outcome and reviewing the arrangements.

The relationship between these three core components is complex: they are not separate but linked in different ways at different times and mutually impinge on one another. Figure 6.1 illustrates the key role played by the care manager in holding together a complex relationship between user/carer and service providers in the context of a fixed budget and other management imperatives.

Essential skills in managing care

While government documents have suggested that a wide range of practitioners from different professional backgrounds and different levels of seniority can be care managers, analysis of the tasks involved indicates the need for a high degree of skill, which practitioners cannot be expected to possess without further training. If care managers are to be catalysts for change, to empower older people and create real choice, then they will need to draw upon a range of skills and also command the authority required to negotiate and secure the best arrangements. The essential skills can be grouped usefully into five categories which are not mutually exclusive but sufficiently distinct to justify separate consideration: interpersonal skills, organizational skills, management skills, creativity and writing skills.

Interpersonal skills include not only the verbal and non-verbal communication skills described in Chapter 4, but also skills of negotiation, bargaining, handling conflict and difference of opinion, establishing personal and professional authority, the ability to challenge constructively and to mediate between others. For example, if an agency can provide only a white domiciliary care worker for an Asian elderly woman, and the service user would prefer an Asian worker, the care manager's role is to negotiate for that service. Such negotiation may involve the need to challenge negative attitudes; to resist the option offered but to keep channels of communication open with the agency; to be prepared to suggest ways in which the preferred option might be secured.

Organizational skills include the ability to organize oneself and other people and involve coordination, team work, the ability to apply a systematic approach, to prioritize tasks and to administer efficiently.

Management skills not only embrace the ability to manage resources but also to manage people, and these are different skills to those of interpersonal communication and organization. Management involves leadership of one kind or another, the ability to take decisions and, in relation to the care manager role, to involve other key people in decision-making in a participative, enabling way. Management skills also include the ability to identify and solve problems, to set objectives, to specify the means by which they can be secured, and to evaluate both process and outcome. Management also refers to the skills required to control and monitor budget and resource allocation and to manage both income and expenditure. Thus, the care manager may not only have to decide on priorities for budget allocation across a number of service users, but also to assess individual service users for their liability to pay charges. Clearly, these tasks demand not only mathematical and financial skills, but the ability to raise and discuss issues which service users may find difficult and which the care manager may wish were not part of her relationship with the user (Lart and Means 1992).

Creativity is essential if the care manager is to be one of the catalysts for the development of new, more flexible services, since this will require practitioners to relinquish the strait-jacket of traditional methods of organizing and delivering services. The approach to domiciliary care, for example, which has tended to provide a 'set menu' of home help and day centre care for people with a wide variety of different needs, must be abandoned if new ways of meeting needs are to be developed. It is extremely difficult to step outside of the context of current conventions and the order of what is familiar, and requires the ability to think laterally and creatively.

Writing skills are extremely important in the process of ensuring that everyone involved in the arrangements understands and agrees precisely what the arrangements are and their own particular role, tasks and functions within the whole. It is also essential that the care manager is able to record the arrangements clearly and in sufficient detail to enable effective monitoring to take place. Experience in other kinds of care provision has shown that unless agreements and care arrangements are recorded systematically in considerable detail (to the degree of defining who does what, and when), the tendency for arrangements to break down is increased. The degree of detail will depend upon the potential for flexibility that can be accommodated by a particular user/carer but may need to specify, for example, the time and day when a particular service will be provided.

The care manager will also need to specify in writing the quality and level of services which are negotiated with providers for particular users. Specification of quality can be difficult to express in writing but must not be avoided if users/carers are to receive the kind of services they need. It is not acceptable if the person who comes to your home to assist you with bathing conducts the process in a manner which is unaffirmative or demeaning. Research has demonstrated consistently that the *way* in which services are delivered, and particularly the personal qualities of the worker, are at least as important a determinant of user satisfaction as the nature or level of service provided (Sainsbury *et al.* 1982; Wilson 1993).

Roles for practitioners in community care

While this chapter has focused upon the role of practitioners as care managers, it is important to locate the care manager role within the context of the spectrum of roles that practitioners may undertake in the provision of community care. There is a danger otherwise that equally important roles become diminished in the professional psyche or that the way in which community care arrangements are implemented will tend to reduce the opportunity for professional helpers to be anything other than care managers. This tendency has been reinforced by the organizational changes within many agencies which have resulted in the separation of commissioning, purchasing and providing roles not only at the level of strategic planning but also at the operational level of service delivery. Many professional helpers have had to face the dilemma of defining themselves, or being defined by senior managers, as either purchasers or providers. In fact, the professional helper is trained to be both and arguably it is in the best interests of user and carers that these key functions remain integrated (Fisher 1991; Huxley 1993). Rigid separation at the operational level may lead to the professional practitioner being designated a purchaser and thereby limited only to assessor and care manager roles. Thus, the potential for direct work with users and carers as part of the package of care would consequently be limited only to that which is consistent with and essential for executing the assessment and care-managing functions (Lamb 1981). The professional helper as counsellor, therapist, provider of skilled interpersonal services, emotional supporter may then not be available as options to older people within community care.

It is therefore essential to locate the role of care manager as one, and only one, of a number of roles which are fundamental to the delivery of professional helping services to older people and their families. Øvretreit (1993: 105) has analysed the 'formal work-role responsibilities' carried by members of a team delivering community care: profession-specific responsibilities; common responsibilities with other team members; case coordination responsibilities.

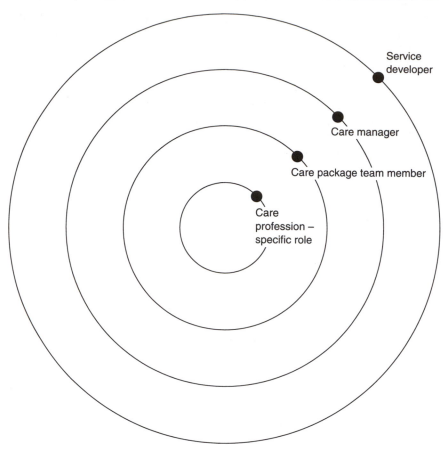

Figure 6.2   Practitioner roles – community care

However, this model can be extended to describe four different roles which practitioners may variously undertake in relation to different users and carers. Adapting Øvretreit's diagrammatic representation, these four roles and their relationship to one another can be conceptualized as four concentric circles (see Fig. 6.2):

- The *core profession-specific role* describes the situation in which the practitioner is caseworker, providing the professional therapeutic help for which he or she is trained, having primary responsibility for assessment and provision of services, although the role and function *vis-à-vis* other professionals will be liaison rather than explicit coordination.
- The role as a *member of the care package team* will include the provision of profession-specific services but in the context of a multidisciplinary network of service providers who, together, constitute the network or package of care. The care package team member is directly accountable not only to the service user/carer for the elements of the care package for which she is

responsible, but also to the other members of the care network and to the care manager.

- As *care manager*, the practitioner may or may not be providing a profession-specific service as part of the care network, but is clearly both a member of the care package team and also responsible for orchestrating, maintaining, monitoring and reviewing the effectiveness of the care package (Renshaw 1988). Thus, the care manager is directly accountable to the service user/carer, to other care package team members for whom she or he has a managerial responsibility, and to the agencies involved jointly in the administration of community care.
- Finally, the practitioner may also have a role to play as *developer of services*, stimulating agencies through the commissioning process to provide what are in short supply or lacking. It is important that the information about unmet needs collated by care managers becomes the catalyst for change and development through the commissioning process (Flynn and Common 1990).

Managing care and anti-discriminatory practice

Much of the official literature about community care has presented the systems for assessment and management of care as value free. The roles, tasks and functions of practitioners have been described in a fairly mechanical way and few of the inherent dilemmas have been discussed. Indeed, one of the inalienable tensions which first appeared in *Caring for People* (DoH 1989a), and has since remained unresolved and largely unacknowledged in government sources, is that between the implementation of a needs-led approach to assessment against a background of limited budgets and resources. It is the care manager who essentially has to face the practical realities and consequences of that tension for individual users and carers.

The issues and dilemmas arising for the care manager will be discussed in detail in the next section. But first it is important to examine the extent to which the care manager may be able to integrate the principles of anti-discriminatory practice within the role, in the light of the seemingly contra-dictory imperatives of meeting need from a pool of services which are limited and, if current trends in local government financing continue, the overall budget for which is likely to decrease. Government publications are instructive on this point: 'The guiding principle of implementation should be to achieve the stated objectives of the care plan with the minimum intervention necessary. It should, therefore, seek to minimise the number of service providers involved' (DoH 1991d: 71). However, practitioners should also be 'tailoring services to individual needs' (p. 14) and 'promoting wider choice' (p. 16).

Add to these contradictory objectives the fact that many older people experience the negative consequences of deep-rooted structural inequalities arising from poverty, race, gender or disability – circumstances over which the care manager has little control – and it is reasonable to predict that the role of care manager may present some threats to the development of anti-discriminatory practice unless it is defined and executed according to principles which, as far as possible, result in enablement and empowerment of the user and carer. The role of care manager has the potential to become either a mechanism for exploitative rationing of insufficient services or the maximization of independence and empowerment of users and carers. Care managers themselves can influence the direction taken in their agencies by attempting to focus their practice on some core anti-discriminatory principles:

- *Centrality of the user and carer*: while this raises its own dilemmas, since not all users are able or equipped to define their needs appropriately or as expansively as they might, the explicit participation of the user/carer and the maximization of choice for them should be a cornerstone of practice (Croft 1992; Beresford and Croft 1994).
- *Support for, not exploitation of, informal support*: users and carers should not be locked into mutually unsatisfactory dependency relationships simply because services are limited.
- *Maximization of quality of life, minimization of risk*: the adoption of these expansive objectives of assessment into the processes of implementation and monitoring will provide important criteria against which the outcome of care packages can be evaluated.
- *Identify inequalities*: the needs of poor or disabled older people, women as users and carers, and people from minority ethnic groups have not been adequately acknowledged or provided for. Care managers will need to link with groups or communities representing disadvantaged older people, press for care managers themselves to be appointed from minority groups and catalyse the development of services which more adequately reflect their needs (NAREA, undated; Franklyn 1992; Blakemore and Boneham 1994).
- *Identify unmet needs*: this is crucial if the care manager's role is to be a force for change and not simply a rationer of scarce resources. To identify unmet need, systematic monitoring and evaluation mechanisms to produce valid and reliable evidence must be set in place.

Issues and dilemmas for the care manager

In this chapter, the roles, tasks and skills inherent in the care manager role have been examined, together with the implications of models of managing care for the development of anti-discriminatory practice. Throughout the discussion, issues and dilemmas which may arise for the care manager during the processes of implementation, monitoring and evaluation have emerged, and this concluding section will summarize those already noted as well as other important issues which must be identified.

The service context

The potential for the care manager role to develop either as 'exploitative rationer' or 'user empowerer' was noted earlier in the chapter. However, there is research evidence which supports the view that, for the care manager to be effective in supporting older people and providing choice, he or she needs the context of a wide range of diverse services upon which to draw. The extent to which a resource-rich service context develops in Britain is a crucial factor in determining the effectiveness of the care manager role.

Accountability

The role involves simultaneous accountability to a number of different constituencies: service users, carers, other professionals, the employing agencies, other agencies, service providers. While accountability to users should be primary for the anti-discriminatory practitioner, in practice the care manager will need to strike a different balance in terms of how these different accountabilities must be exercised in different cases and situations.

Conflict and difference

A key element in the role is the ability to predict, negotiate and constructively challenge and mediate conflict, conflicts of interest and different opinions about what should or should not be done (Payne 1986). This is a characteristic of all multidisciplinary teamwork and many practitioners will be familiar with and skilled in the management of conflict and difference. However, a crucial factor is the status of the care manager and how she or he is perceived, particularly by other professionals in different agencies. For example, a community nurse acting as care manager may have increased difficulty managing differences with a general practitioner or the senior manager of a social services department, not because she is unskilled but because the attitude of professionals who regard themselves as higher-ranking may negatively influence the negotiation process. As Biegel *et al.* (1984: 94) perceptively commented, 'Everyone wants to coordinate but no-one wants to be coordinated'.

Responsibility without power

A related issue for the care manager is responsibility for the management of the care package without executive management responsibility for the people delivering the services. Having responsibility for implementation and outcome without having the power to manage the elements within the package constitutes an important break in the normal linkage between responsibility and power and may cause considerable dilemmas for care managers.

The unwilling client

The assumptions underpinning the community care arrangements portray a picture of service users who want and need services and who are ready and able to cooperate with professional helpers in the identification of need and provision of services. Fisher (1990a, 1990b, 1990c) and others (Levin *et al.* 1988; Huxley 1993) have made an important contribution to the debate concerning the arrangements for implementing community care. They have raised the question of how far the models for assessment and care managing, with the attendant organizational changes towards purchaser and provider separation, are compatible with the roles and functions the professional helper must undertake with people who are either unwilling or unable to define their own needs and engage with the helping process. Fisher (1990a) also challenges the relevance of the concept and language of consumerism, which is the cornerstone of the underlying assumptions behind the community care arrangements: that the creation of a facsimile of the market is the most effective means of ensuring 'consumer' supremacy. While 'care managers will need to uphold the rights of each party to be treated as a competent adult' (Fisher 1990a: 225), enshrining those rights in practice presents major obstacles when, for example, the user is an elderly person with severe dementia. Huxley (1993) pursues this theme and argues that the 'administrative model of case management' fails to acknowledge such dilemmas and obscures the need for professional judgement to be exercised, not in an unaccountable or unthinking manner but with sensitivity and from the perspective of an advocate. The role of professional judgement must remain at the heart of managing care if the care manager is to be able to meet and, if possible, resolve some of the difficult human dilemmas which community care presents.

Managing risk

Finally, the role of the care manager through time inherently involves the monitoring and management of risk. While the assessor is responsible for describing and evaluating the nature and level of risk, it is the care manager who must attempt to minimize and contain risk through the provision of services. This involves continuing monitoring, evaluation and reassessment, especially when circumstances or conditions change. It also involves the balancing of rights with risk and, often, the containment of other people's anxieties when the risks are perceived by them to be high. Not least, the care manager has to carry her own concerns about levels of risk and should seek and receive support in so doing.

7

Direct work with users and carers

Paradoxically, community care, as defined, evidences a migration away from direct contact between elders and practitioners.

(Biggs 1993: 143)

Biggs (1993) and others (Fisher 1991; Huxley 1993) have identified the means by which a particular model of the community care process tends to reduce the opportunity for health and social service practitioners to provide direct services themselves. As noted in the previous chapter, much of the official literature has defined an *administrative* model of community care which implicitly limits the role of practitioners to assessing need and arranging services provided by other people. The role of the care manager, in particular, is seen as essentially technical and administrative, managing the interface between user choice and resource availability. The care manager role *vis-à-vis* the user within this model is one of *ensuring provision*. While the care manager will need to use professional skills to assist the user to articulate preferences and negotiate with providers to secure the best-fit services to meet need and demand, the care manager has not generally been defined as a potential provider herself. Indeed, the concept of the care package within this model rarely includes services designed to address emotional, psychological or relationship problems, but seems to have returned to a 'welfare' model of care which defines older people's needs in terms of practical support and aids to living. It has been a major theme throughout this book that such a reduced and over-simplified view of older people is a reflection of pervasive ageist attitudes, and other chapters have sought to demonstrate how practitioners can attempt to develop a more sensitive, elaborative view of their roles through the assessment and care management procedures. However, it is also essential that practitioners continue to define themselves, and their colleagues, as potential providers of the kind of services for which they are trained and from which some older people would benefit. Discussion of the administrative model of community care and an alternative model which endorses professional expertise will be developed in the final chapter.

Another notable feature of community care procedures is the relative emphasis upon the care manager's role *vis-à-vis* different and competing constituencies: user, carer, provider agencies. There is a danger that, in attempting to secure care services from both carer and other agencies, particularly in a situation in which care options may be limited, the care manager's job *in practice* will involve more contact with informal and formal carers and less contact with service users.

Finally, and focusing in particular on the general requirement that community care arrangements emphasize equally the needs of carers and are designed, first and foremost, to enable family and informal carers to continue caring, the institutionalization of informal carers as primary components of the care package runs the risk of elevating the importance of carers' needs and obscuring the distinct and separate needs of elderly users. Biggs (1993: 144) summarizes the cumulative effect of these characteristics of community care arrangements as follows:

> At each point, the possibility of collusive alliances between generational peers . . . may marginalise the existential needs of older people themselves. A trend, noted at various points in the caring system, works towards homogenization of elders as a group, denies the role of . . . and conflict between perspectives, and theory obscures the reality of these users' perspectives with results that closely follow commonly held prejudices against elders. The practice of community care, it would seem, produces a new form of institutionalised ageism.

It is for this reason that a chapter on direct work with users and carers is included as an essential component of a book about community care. However, within the limitations of a single chapter, the potential for considering the full range of practice methods which may be applicable to the needs of older people cannot be realized and therefore it has been necessary to select a small number of practice methods to illustrate how these might be applied. The methods included are both those which have been most closely associated with work with elders, such as reminiscence, and others such as family-focused work, which has not generally been used with older people as service users. The chapter examines work with individuals, work with families and groups and, finally, considers a number of special issues in work with older people.

Working with individuals

There is no method of therapeutic practice that cannot be applied to work with older people provided, as with clients of other ages, the method selected is appropriate to the abilities and wishes of the user, the experience of the worker and the nature of the identified problem. The difficulty for practitioners is that much of the literature which has developed the theory and practice of therapeutic work has not included older people, for instance, in case studies and has not discussed the issues which need to be taken into account in applying the method to work with older people. In short, older people it would seem are noticeable only by their absence within the bulk of literature on therapeutic methods and therefore have, by default, been defined as inappropriate subjects for therapeutic help. It is little wonder that professionals working with older people have struggled to develop a range of therapeutic methods which have been tested and evaluated with older people. Nevertheless, there is no reason in principle why a task-centred approach, crisis intervention, psychotherapeutic work, behavioural approaches, among others, cannot be useful in helping older people in appropriate circumstances. The methods of work which are considered here are reminiscence and counselling.

Reminiscence, personal biography and life review therapy

The subject of reminiscence and whether it has special significance for older people is fraught with difficulty and confusion, both conceptually and in terms of the extent to which some form of remembering or re-evaluating past life can be applied therapeutically within a professional helping relationship (Molinari and Reichlin 1985). In part, the confusion is a product of the chequered history of reminiscence within academic and professional thinking and reflects an attempt, which has not yet been wholly successful, to rehabilitate the concept of reminiscence from that of the ramblings of increasingly confused old people to an ordinary, functional activity, common throughout all age groups, which may have special application in therapeutic work with old people. However, a considerable lack of clarity remains about how reminiscence should be conceptualized and applied in practice, and what its benefits are to older service users (Norris 1986). It is also true that work of dubious quality, particularly in groups, has been conducted with older people on the basis of an inadequate understanding of the issues involved and the values which must underpin such work if it is to avoid oppressive practice (Harris and Hopkins 1994). This will be discussed in a later section on groupwork.

While people of all ages appear to want, at times, to look back and tell stories about their earlier lives – and indeed the extent to which parents and care agencies can tell stories about the past is regarded as crucially important to a child's sense of identity – it is the storytelling by older people which has tended to be called 'reminiscence' and embued with negative connotations associated with mental deterioration, living in the past and a process of disengaging from the mainstream of life (Scrutton 1989). Coleman (1994) has argued that, contrary to accepted wisdom, the emergence of disengagement theory, which legitimized introspection as a natural and inevitable consequence of old age, also marked the beginning of a more positive view of reminiscence. In fact, disengagement theory, as Chapter 1 has argued, legitimized a view of older people which, overall, was negative in so far as it depicted old age as a time of withdrawal and disengagement. Consequently, disengagement theory validated a construction of older people which emphasized passivity and retrospection and linked reminiscence with that construction as the primary means by which the present was relinquished.

Thus, reminiscence became a process firmly associated with older people and, moreover, with a generally negative view of old age. The link was consolidated when Butler (1963) outlined a theory that the 'life review' is a normative process, undertaken as people approach the end of life, and essential to the achievement of acceptance of self before death intervenes. 'Reminiscence' and 'life review' became connected but in ways which lacked definitional clarity. The terms were used interchangeably and the general benefits of the normal process of life review – self-esteem, psychological health and integration (Erikson 1982) – were also assumed to apply to reminiscence. Finally, the concept of life review as a structured therapeutic process has been added to the debate. The definition and terminology now embraces reminiscence, life review, life history, personal biography and life review therapy and the debate is now characterized by some fundamental thematic questions:

- Is reminiscence an 'ordinary activity' or a 'specialized activity' requiring expert guidance?
- Does the concept of reminiscence enhance a positive, anti-ageist view of older people or does it tend to confirm negative stereotypes?
- What is the value of reminiscence to individuals in general and older people in particular?
- What is the value of reminiscence to society?

It would be more helpful if the term 'reminiscence' was expunged from theoretical and professional vocabulary, overladen as it is with contradictory definitions and concepts. In developing a model for conceptualizing what could be called 'recall activity', it is reasonable to expect that recall can take place on different levels, be spontaneous or catalysed, free-flowing or structured, spasmodic or planned, alone or with assistance, and be part of everyday activity or a therapeutic relationship. Thus 'recalling the past' involves a spectrum of activities ranging from the spontaneous recounting of brief stories or episodes, possibly prompted by a picture or event, to the systematic recall and evaluation of the chronological sequences of experiences through which a life has progressed. All may be used by professional helpers, but each particular level of recall activity is probably best suited to different therapeutic objectives and it is important that methods are linked clearly to appropriate objectives.

For the purpose of clarifying the range of activities associated with recall, the spectrum can be conceptualized as consisting of three main types of recall activity (see Table 7.1). There is inevitably overlap between these three levels of activity, described here as storytelling, personal biography (or life history) and life review therapy. All have therapeutic applications and can be linked to a range of objectives for worker and older person, from relationship building through to facilitating a troubled older person facing unresolved conflicts or death. Figure 7.1 illustrates how the three different levels of recall activity may be appropriately linked to different levels of practitioner–user objectives.

Storytelling – and listening – can be a particularly useful means of bridging the age difference between younger helper and older person and thereby of establishing trust and confidence within the relationship. It is also important as a means of acknowledging the different experiences – and therefore values –

Table 7.1 The spectrum of recall activity

Storytelling	Personal biography	Life review therapy
Spontaneous	Catalysed	Catalysed
Free-flowing	Structured	Structured
Spasmodic	Planned	Planned
Recall of snapshots	Recall of life	Recall of life
Descriptive	Descriptive	Evaluative
Focus on social history	Focus on personal strengths	Focus on past difficulties

which may characterize the respective perspectives of worker and user. However, the recounting of extracts from personal history is also crucial for the validation of the personal identity of the older person and therefore for understanding more completely the complexity of the older individual (Johnson 1976; Coleman 1986; Tobin 1991). Validation arises through two means. First, stories from the past confirm the older person as the product of a much more valid range of experiences than perhaps his or her current circumstances might suggest: the older person is, if you like, the tip of a vast experiential iceberg, most of which is hidden from contemporary eyes. Thus, the depth of *personal history* is a crucial validating factor. Second, however, the older person is the repository of knowledge and experience of *social history*

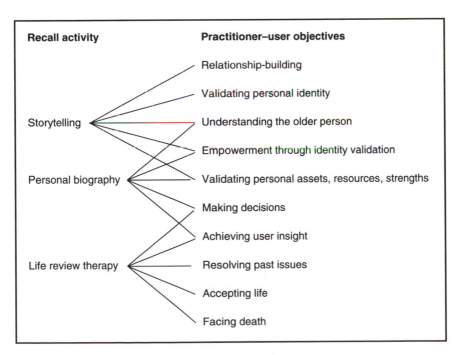

Figure 7.1 Linking recall activity to therapeutic objectives

which is of profound importance to community and societal identity. To be able to talk about life in another era with its momentous events such as war confers importance upon older people. Finally, through personal validation, the older person may begin to feel in control of the current situation, even if the storytelling is not specifically structured to achieve this outcome.

Personal biography work is similar to life history work undertaken with children and young people when they move from one placement to another or in a more general way when there is a need to confirm and enhance a child's sense of identity. It is the structured reconstruction of the chronological events through which a person has passed, and designed to record not only the events and the facts, but also the feelings with which they were accompanied. While the personal biography will inevitably identify negative experiences and past difficulties, the objective of the work is to articulate the strengths, resources and qualities the individual has already demonstrated in moving through those periods and arriving in the present. Thus, personal biography work is designed to produce a record – factual and emotional – of a person's life, to applaud that life and, through the process of work, to enable the individual to meet challenges in the *present situation* (Coleman 1994).

Thus, personal biography can address a range of objectives including understanding and empowerment, validating personal strengths, decision-making and enabling users to begin to evaluate the extent to which past strengths can be applied to current problems. It may begin to resolve past conflicts or issues but is not necessarily designed to do so without specific psychotherapeutic guidance from the practitioner.

Life review therapy, on the other hand, is closer to Butler's concept of addressing the challenges of the past in order to accept one's life and thereby face death (Garland 1994). The primary focus is upon the development of insight through processes of analysis and evaluation of past events, to formulate an acceptance of past difficulties, which includes a degree of resolution and which thereby includes a psychological quiescence in the face of approaching death. Life review therapy, therefore, is a variant of psychotherapeutic counselling directed at problems in the past which may be inhibiting the achievement of ego integrity or, put more simply, the acceptance of one's life and all its features (Butler 1974).

The *practice methods* by which recall authority is introduced into direct work will depend on the practitioner-worker objectives and the level of recall activity which most appropriately facilitates those objectives. However, as with service users from other groups, the use of materials and aids as a vehicle for recall is usually helpful. Storytelling, for example, can be triggered by and developed from a photograph. Personal biography and life review therapy, however, may utilize a range of techniques, including scrapbooks, collecting items, revisiting places, writing, audiotaping or videotaping an autobiography, photograph albums, diaries, family genealogy, talking into a mirror or guided imagery (Beaver 1991; Garland 1994) and furthermore requires the skills of the worker to assist with analysis and evaluation (Merriman 1989).

A number of issues for practice arise when personal biography or life review therapy is undertaken:

- *Preparation*: the practitioner must prepare extensively for the work, and this includes preparation of the user and of self. The practitioner must be aware that the process may make practical and emotional demands on both worker and user, particularly when painful experiences are recounted.
- *Avoiding assumptions*: both personal biography and life review therapy involve the charting of feelings, not just facts. However, the worker must consciously avoid suggesting or predicting the feelings that might have accompanied a particular event and instead be careful to elicit from the user the actual feelings experienced. For example, an assumption that the early death of a father resulted in grief and unhappiness may make it impossible for an elderly woman to disclose the guilt and relief she felt when her father's death brought to an end long-standing child abuse.
- *Open-ended questions*: avoiding assumptions implies the conscious use of open-ended questions to explore experiences and the feelings which accompanied them.
- *Confronting painful memories*: life biography and life review therapy will inevitably reveal events which were not only painful at the time but whose memory revives the painful feelings and emotions in the present. It is important that the worker does not shrink back from hearing these experiences and sharing the emotions, although to do so can be difficult, especially for the practitioner who is anxious to 'solve problems' in a practical way.
- *Finding positive memories*: equally important within the process is the retrieval of positive memories of events which endorse the qualities and strengths of the individual (Coleman 1994).

Storytelling, personal biography and life review therapy are forms of recall activity which are linked to the development of a strong sense of identity, self-esteem and psychological health (Tobin 1991). In working with individuals, practitioners must be clear about the reasons for using recall activity, define the objectives of work and assess with the older person the level of recall activity to be employed, the form it will take and the time-scale involved.

A major advantage of recall activity arises from the emergence of facets of life which are inextricably connected to personal characteristics of class, gender, race, disability and sexuality (Hughes and Mtezuka 1992). The personal biography of a woman or a black elder, for example, will speak not only of the experiences of that person as a unique human being, but also as a person whose life has, in part, been constructed by social and political attitudes to the group – women, black people – which to some extent they represent (Blakemore 1985). This presents particular challenges, for example, to a young white male practitioner who must take account of such user–practitioner differences and consider the impact they may have on the recall activity. However, recall activity also offers a particularly effective way for the practitioner to understand as empathetically as possible the impact of institutionalized discrimination, the ways in which individuals negotiated and, at a micro level, transcended discrimination, and the connection between these experiences and their views, expectations and values in old age.

Counselling

Counselling embraces a wide range of approaches based on a number of different theoretical constructs (Coulshed 1988). However, a common feature of much of the literature on counselling is the absence of elderly people from case material used to illustrate how and in what situations different counselling models can be applied. Scrutton (1989), whose book is a significant challenge to the apparent belief among counsellors that older people and their problems are not suitable or interesting subjects, cites the pervasive influence of ageism as the primary reason. The neglect of older people within counselling theory and practice implies that older people's needs are comparatively simple and easily satisfied, usually by the provision of practical aids. Alternatively, 'there may also be an assumption that counselling older people is essentially similar to counselling any other age group' (Scrutton 1989: 9), but as Scrutton points out, there are special considerations to be taken into account in any form of direct work with older people, including counselling. A major theme of this book has been to challenge the over-simplified, homogeneous view of older people which reflects ageist values. Practitioners must maintain a careful balance between practice which does not pathologize unnecessarily older people whose needs *are* simple, while at the same time being open to the possibility that some older people have complex, emotional or relationship problems which packages of practical services alone cannot address. A knowledge of counselling and its associated skills must be part of the repertoire of the practitioner working with older people.

What is counselling?

It is beyond the scope of this chapter to provide a detailed analysis and evaluation of the range of perspectives and methods which are included within counselling. The reader wishing to develop counselling skills with older people should pursue the references included here as a starting point for research. The intention in this section is to provide a summary of the definitions, skills and objectives of counselling and some of the strengths and limitations of its application to work with older people.

Counselling is fundamentally concerned with a relationship between counsellee and counsellor in that 'the quality of the counselling depends on the quality of the relationship' (Scrutton 1989: 46). Skills are important, but the relationship as the medium for work is fundamental. Scrutton identifies three key aspects of counselling: a relationship, skills and a process of personal development. Rogers (1951a, 1951b) and Egan (1981) have each elaborated different models of counselling, the former advocating a 'client-centred' approach and the latter a 'problem-solving' approach. Psychotherapeutic models are based on Freudian theory and will not be discussed here, as they are based on quite different principles and a different concept of the worker–older person relationship.

Most counselling approaches are based on a number of principles which define the purpose, methods and, in particular, the attitudes which should underpin the practitioner role:

• non-judgemental attitude

- unconditional positive regard
- empathetic understanding
- genuineness
- trust
- confidentiality

However, some of these principles can be difficult to implement in practice with older people. For example, empathetic understanding may be difficult to achieve to the same degree as with other clients, not least because practitioners will usually have no experience of old age – it is part of their future, not their past or present. Paradoxically, attempting to work in an anti-oppressive way may complicate the achievement of unconditional positive regard with older people. The ability to recognize the victimization of older people as a group by society may tend to lead to a view of individual older people as inherently victims too. A victim-only perspective can make it difficult to acknowledge that some older people, as people of any age, are difficult to engage, have unpleasant personalities or problematic behaviour. Practitioners may thus attempt to counsel older people for whom they do not have genuine positive regard. Counselling under such circumstances is unlikely to be productive.

A victim-only perspective can also contaminate the *process* of counselling, which includes not only listening, interpreting, hypothesizing, confirming and clarifying, but also challenging. Challenging may involve posing alternative understandings or explanations for current difficulties, identifying when the process of counselling has become stuck or presenting the conflicting perspective of a significant other. Challenge may include saying things which the older person will not want to hear. To be able to challenge, the practitioner must have confidence in her skills, and hold on to the principles underlying the process but not allow a 'victim-only perspective' or a fear of upsetting an older person to be reasons for avoiding necessary challenge. To do so is to dehumanize older people. Hashimi (1991) goes further and identifies three common ways in which practitioners, often benignly or unconsciously, violate the norms of good counselling practice:

- *Overprotection*: a failure to challenge; completing the task on behalf of the user; over-control of the process.
- *Anything goes*: a failure to challenge; a view that the principles of self-determination and non-judgemental attitude preclude practitioner opinions on the inadvisability, destructiveness or risks of certain behaviours.
- *Insensitivity*: a failure to interpret behaviour or meaning accurately arising from a lack of knowledge of older people and their experiences.

Purposes of counselling
Counselling can be applied to a wide range of issues facing many elder people: bereavement, loss of functional ability, relationship conflict or difficulty, connecting the past with the present, understanding and changing current circumstances, adaptation to new circumstances, assessing personal needs, managing stress and working through distress. Counselling skills will also be applied not only in similar therapeutic processes, such as personal biography and life review therapy, but also during procedures which are not of

themselves therapeutic but with which counselling *skills* can assist (Nelson-Jones 1983). For example, the gathering of information to assess or elicit a user's degree of satisfaction with a care package as part of quality assurance will draw upon counselling skills. The purposes, or main outcomes, of counselling are the achievement of understanding or change, making decisions, resolving intrapersonal conflicts, improving relationships or assimilating and coming to terms with difficult experiences.

Working with families

The emphasis within community care on the needs and wishes of carers inevitably directs the practitioner towards a focus upon the family as well as the older person (Froggatt 1990). Whether or not family members undertake a caring role *vis-à-vis* the elderly person, one of the main dilemmas for practitioners in family-focused work is the balancing of the needs, interests and views of different family members. Not only may these be different, they may be in conflict and, if so, the practitioner must execute considerable sensitivity and skill in finding a way through. Perhaps one of the most acute conflicts of interests occurs when, in the face of increasing dependency or after hospitaliz-ation, the older person wishes to return home, but other family members prefer the older person to relinquish home and either move in with a relative or enter residential care. If, in returning home, the elderly person is dependent upon these same family members for support, the conflict of interest inherent in the decision-making process is clearly apparent. In most cases such as this, the wishes of the elderly person may be accommodated with support services, although the anxiety of the family members will not necessarily be assuaged. However, in other situations the conflicts of interest are more subtle and complex and difficult to unravel. For example, an adult daughter who wants to continue caring for her elderly mother may need respite care to be able to do so, but the older person may refuse to stay for even short periods with her son (with whom she has never got on) and be equally resistant to attending a day centre. Creative ways may be found to meet both sets of needs, but a solution will depend in part on the options available and the sensitivity and negotiating skills of the practitioner.

This raises the related issue of the role of the practitioner *vis-à-vis* different family members: advocate for the older person; advocate for the carer; neutral facilitator? Scrutton (1989) argues that the practitioner must demonstrate neutrality, otherwise credibility will be undermined. However, power differ-entials within families mean that not all members are equally equipped to engage in a shared counselling or decision-making process and thus the practitioner must assist a particular, less powerful person when necessary. Older people are likely, but not inevitably, to be less powerful. Parents can continue to dominate children even in adulthood and relationship patterns of this kind often persist even when caring roles are reversed.

Issues in family-focused work

- *Who comprises the family?* Changes in social behaviour through divorce and the reconstitution of second families have resulted in a greater variety of more extended families than in the past. An elderly person may have had more than one long-term partnership, each of which has produced children. The adult children of an older person may also have children by different partners, producing different generations of grandchildren. In limited families, an unmarried elderly woman might regard distant nieces as her closest family. In a very extended, complex family, the person closest emotionally to an elderly person may not be the closest generationally. Particularly in decisions about the future, the elderly person may confer upon some relatives the right to be involved, but exclude others. *Who* should decide who is in the family for purposes such as these?

- *Age and circumstances of carers.* In some instances, carers themselves may be elderly, for example a 73-year-old woman caring for her 82-year-old brother. Alternatively, a married daughter may be caught in an inter-generational caring trap, with dependent children and dependent parents.
- *Family history.* Family secrets, relationships, rules, roles of individuals and the history of family dynamics will have an important impact on family-focused work.
- *Power differentials.* In part these will derive from age and current social, economic and personal circumstances, but will also be a reflection of the history of power differentials within a particular family. The older person may be more or less powerful than other people but will often be relatively powerless. Factors such as gender, class and race will also influence how power differentials are evidenced in different families.
- *Ability and motivation to engage.* The older person and relevant family members have to be both functionally able and motivated for family-focused work to be undertaken. Functional disabilities which impair communication effectively disempower a person, for example, and must be overcome if family interviews are to take place.

Purposes of family-focused work

Scrutton (1989: 92) describes family work as a 'cooperative problem-solving process that the family undertakes with the worker' and defines the primary task as the illumination of 'the different view points of key members of the family group, how they differ from each other and why stress in family relationships has developed'. However, family-focused work is not only applicable to problems *within* the family, but also to problems between the family and the wider system. The practitioner must assess with the older person and the family the nature and location of the problem and this should help the practitioner to decide how to proceed. For example, relationship difficulties may be addressed by initially talking about family history, whereas an external problem facing the family as a unit may require a task-centred approach focused on the present.

Methods of work

It is helpful to distinguish two broad approaches to family-focused work with older people: family counselling and family therapy. Family counselling takes the principles and skills of counselling and applies them to family groups. It may or may not see the family as a system, but it does not apply rigorously the principles of system theory. The focus instead is a humanist perspective which attempts, through counselling and negotiation skills, to resolve problems and enable individuals in the family to develop. Therefore, it can readily embrace issues of power differentials which derive both from established patterns of relationships and from sources of structural inequality. Family therapy, on the other hand, is based upon a systemic view of the family, in which individuals are components and in which it is the *interactions* between individuals which are the focus of attention. The *characteristics* of individuals are considered less important. Family therapy has been criticized for its failure to accommodate issues of power differentials, although some of the skills developed by family therapists – circular questioning, positive reframing – can be usefully applied in family-focused work.

Working with groups

While there has been some development of groupwork with carers of older people in Britain, it is to the American literature we must turn for examples of the diverse ways in which groupwork can be used with older people themselves (e.g. National Association of Social Workers 1963; Klein *et al.* 1965; Burnside 1978; Silverstone and Burack-Weiss 1983; Hancock 1987; MacLennan *et al.* 1988). In Britain, groupwork is not often used with older people unless they are confused or in a setting such as residential or day care where they are, in a sense, a 'captive' group. However, even with these particular categories of older people, groupwork has in general been limited to an organized activity focused upon reminiscence or craft work.

Harris and Hopkins (1994: 75), in an analysis of reminiscence groupwork, 'question the extent to which much of the group-based reminiscence in residential and day-care settings may be seen as providing an adequate conceptual and practice foundation for anti-discriminatory practice with older people'. Many of the groups they observed had been conducted by students on placement or by junior members of staff untrained in groupwork. Sessions tended to be based on the routinized use of reminiscence kits, consisting of cards, slides, videos, posters or artefacts, to stimulate discussion. The purpose of such groups was often ill-defined and tended to reflect a vague notion that allowing elderly people to talk about the past in some way validates their personal histories, empowers them and, therefore, is an example of anti-discriminatory practice. However, given the way in which such groups have been conducted (e.g. their membership decided by staff; little consideration of whether the members of the group have sufficient shared history, particularly when there may be twenty years difference in age and different class and cultural backgrounds; lack of knowledge and skill on the part of workers; lack of clarity about purpose and process and the extensive use of pre-packaged kits), 'organized reminiscence groups ... run the danger of implicitly reinforcing ageist attitudes toward older people by confirming a view of them as conservative, preoccupied with personal memories and collective expressions of nostalgia' (Harris and Hopkins 1994: 82), and for whom more

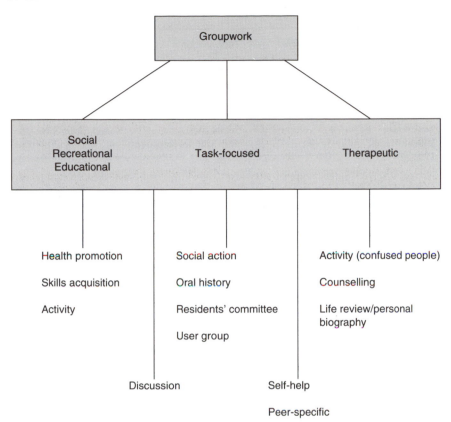

Figure 7.2 A conceptual model of groupwork with older people

rigorous or specific groupwork is inappropriate. The purpose of this section is to extend conventional thinking beyond organized reminiscence groups to consider how a range of different types of groupwork may be employed with older people and carers.

Conceptualizing groupwork

A number of models for conceptualizing groupwork have been proposed (for a summary and typology of six models, see Brown 1986), although few British writers have considered the special issues involved in working with groups of older people. Drawing upon the general groupwork literature and the American social work literature, the framework in Fig. 7.2 offers a model for conceptualizing groupwork possibilities with both older people and their carers. At one end of the spectrum are groups whose primary activity is social, educational or recreational. Other groups may be explicitly focused upon a task, function or campaign, while at the other end of the spectrum are groups whose activity is explicitly therapeutic and concerned with the personal development of the individual members.

Table 7.2   Types of groups and their purposes

	Social/recreational/ educational	Task-focused	Therapeutic
Primary purpose	Social interaction, skill enhancement, functional maintenance	Task achievement, skill enhancement	Personal development, therapeutic change
Secondary purpose	Personal development	Social interaction, personal development	Social interaction

There are a number of purposes, or objectives, of groupwork: social interaction, skill enhancement, functional maintenance, task achievement, personal development and therapeutic change. Each type of group activity is more closely connected with some of these purposes than with others, although all groups address most of these objectives in one way or another. It is helpful to conceptualize each type of group activity as having a set of primary purposes with which it is most closely linked, but acknowledging also the secondary purposes which can be identified. Table 7.2 summarizes the primary and secondary purposes associated with each kind of group activity and also illustrates the overlap which inevitably exists between them.

It is possible to use this model to define a particular kind of group, its primary and secondary purposes and thereby prepare, plan, implement and evaluate the group in a systematic way. For example, a keep-fit group with lucid older people may be established as a recreational group whose primary purposes are functional maintenance (keeping fit) and social interaction. However, a keep-fit class for older confused people may be used to address some issues of personal development, as the exercises are designed primarily to preserve or improve brain–body coordination and engender a sense of control and, thereby, esteem. Thus a keep-fit group for confused older people might have an explicit therapeutic purpose.

The model also helps to conceptualize the different forms of recall activity upon which groups can be based: an oral history group established to chart and record social history and its connection with personal lives is essentially task-focused, with possible secondary benefits to some group members through social interaction and personal development through group participation. However, use of personal biography or life review as a therapeutic process involves a group with a very different purpose, which would require quite different planning, rules, interpretation skills and criteria for evaluation. The critical issue for practitioners is to be clear about the type of group, its activities and purposes and to ensure that these are appropriately linked.

The benefits of different kinds of groupwork with older people have not been systematically evaluated and there is a dearth of practice experience upon which to draw. The American literature, however, does include a number of evaluative studies which variously claim positive outcomes, including increased social interaction, confidence, emotional support, affirmation of identity, restoration of diminished roles and functions, maintenance of physical and mental faculties, education, opportunities for reflection, problem-solving and general improvement (Rose 1991).

Issues in establishing a user or carer group

A number of issues need to be considered when setting up a group for older people and some of these also apply to carers.

Composition and membership. The rule of thumb in groupwork theory is to aim for a membership in which individuals are sufficiently homogeneous on key criteria to be able to relate to each other but sufficiently heterogeneous to stimulate interest and active engagement. Reference has already been made to the ageist tendency to see older people as a homogeneous group, despite considerable differences in age, social history, class, gender, race, sexuality and levels of ability. Every age cohort of elderly people is highly heterogeneous. Thus the criteria for commonality between group members has to be considered carefully and the degree and types of difference need to be managed in different ways for different groups. In general, groups which involve less intimate interaction will tolerate greater heterogeneity than those in which personal disclosure is a feature. There may also be differences in the extent to which confused elderly people can accommodate difference, given the demands upon their impaired mental functioning, and it has been argued that when older people are very frail, especially mentally, a greater degree of homogeneity among members assists the group process. Racial origin and cultural background are also criteria which ought to be **given** specific consideration, as should gender for some groups.

Boundary. Is it more appropriate for a particular group to be open or closed? Is it time-limited or indefinite?

Ground rules. What rules do the members need to agree about confidentiality and the behaviour of members towards one another? What is the agreed purpose of the group?

Leadership. Some groups may be peer-led or practitioner-led. The role of the leader in most groups is crucial, and if he or she is a practitioner, the leader must be clear about the role involved, and this will be dependent upon the kind of group established and the characteristics of its members. In any group, the leader must undertake preparation, monitor and review the group sessions and evaluate the effectiveness of the group over time.

Practical issues. Venue is important for some types of groupwork with older people, or carers, and the quality of the environment may be a significant factor in facilitating group process. However, the organization of transport is often a considerable problem, especially for older people with disabilities, and groups for older people will flounder unless this practical issue can be addressed and reliable transport arranged.

Special issues in direct work

The purpose of this section is to draw attention to a number of issues which are important in direct work with older people and their families, either because they tend to arise frequently or because, conversely, they are issues which are often neglected or unrecognized.

Dependency

Many older people who are referred to health and social service practitioners are physically or mentally disabled, or both. Ageist attitudes assume that old age is synonymous with disability, despite evidence that this is not the case. However, by definition, older people who need services are experiencing problems of living and many of these are due to a disability which, in turn, creates a dependency on some form of family, informal or formal support. The impact of dependency may be three-fold: self-image, role-reversal and user/carer conflict.

Biographical accounts of older people have testified to a common experience of becoming old: the disjunction between the image of the inner self and the bodily image (Matthews 1979; Ford and Sinclair 1987; Biggs 1993). Older people often do not describe themselves as old and report that they do not *feel* old (Thompson 1992). They feel inside exactly the same as they did in middle-age or younger. However, they have somehow to link that inner self with the old self which is seen both in the mirror and in the reactions of other people. It may be argued that the disjunction only exists because Western society does not value old bodies and therefore older people themselves are reproducing ageist attitudes when they identify with the still-young inner self but not the old bodily self. However, we each internalize to a degree social constructions of our particular characteristics, and practitioners should not expect older people alone to be able to stand outside powerful social norms. The disjunction *is* experienced by many older people and, indeed, is strained further when the body not only looks old but ceases to function normally.

Dependency also changes social and personal roles when a formerly independent person, one who may have been a carer of others, becomes cared-for. Role-reversal not only has to be accommodated psychologically by the older person but it may also challenge relationships. Finally, as this chapter has already identified, the user–carer relationship constructed upon dependency is highly complex and, while many such relationships are harmonious, they may be liable to develop both conflict and conflict of interest. The relationship is constructed as dependent–independent rather than one of mutual interdependence (Morris 1992).

Confusion and dementia

Confused behaviour in older people can be caused by a variety of factors, of which dementia is only one:

- Illness or infection, particularly those which cause a rise in temperature such as a urinary infection, can cause temporary confusion.
- Iatrogenic intervention (i.e. the administration of a drug, or more usually a cocktail of drugs) can produce a confusional state. Again, the effect is temporary.

- Biological disorders – for example, a hormone imbalance, possibly due to a malfunction in specific organs such as the liver or kidney, can be accompanied by a confusional state.
- Poor nutrition, resulting in deficiencies in vitamins or minerals, has been linked with confused behaviour.
- Social factors (e.g. bereavement, loss, unexpected trauma) precipitate distress which not only has a psychological effect, but may stimulate biochemical reactions and the release of substances which alter the brain's capacity to function.
- Multi-infarct dementia: the narrowing of arteries to the brain reduces the blood supply and causes blockages, resulting in a series of small strokes, or haemorrhages, which often go unnoticed, but which gradually destroy brain cells. As deterioration progresses, or in the event of more significant strokes which destroy discernible parts of the brain, loss of physical and mental function occurs. Although the damage itself is irreparable, the progress of the condition can be characterized by partial recovery of function after each stroke, although the overall pattern over a period of years is one of gradual brain death and loss of function. The pattern, however, will vary considerably from one person to another and be dependent upon how frequently and where localized damage occurs.
- Alzheimer's disease: this is a gradual degeneration of brain cells through an unknown cause. Onset and progress is gradual initially, but proceeds towards further degeneration without remission or partial recovery. However, the pace at which degeneration occurs varies considerably, with some individuals progressing rapidly towards very severe impairment, while others may remain only mildly confused for some time. The effects of the illness are currently permanent and irreversible and lead eventually to death if no other illness intervenes.

The signs of confusion vary according to the cause and, in the case of a progressive condition, the extent of degeneration. Mild, temporary confused behaviour may consist of disorientation in time or place, disturbance of speech, loss of ability to take care of oneself, hearing voices or paranoia. Alzheimer's disease results in progressive brain damage which follows a pattern, attacking initially parts of the brain which control peripheral functions and progressing to the core functions which sustain life itself. Thus, the changes in behaviour also tend to follow a loose pattern, beginning with short-term memory loss and speech disturbance progressing to disinhibition in social behaviour, loss of coordination, loss of speech, hallucinations, and eventually major loss of muscle function and control. However, although the disease may be due to brain degeneration, the *impact* of the illness on behaviour is mediated by the degree to which environmental characteristics are either sympathetic or hostile to the loss of function (Kitwood and Bredin 1992).

Direct work with confused people must be based upon extensive knowledge of the causes of confusion and the progress of degenerative conditions (Marshall 1993). In the early stages, older people may be very aware of their impaired cognitive functioning and this can lead to depression which often goes unrecognized and untreated. Work must be based upon explicit anti-ageist values, without which it is all too easy to depersonalize the confused older person. Three main methods of work have been developed: reality orientation, validation therapy and reminiscence (or recall activity).

Reality orientation seeks to maintain the confused older person in the real world by continually reinforcing reality while at the same time either ignoring or actively challenging confused behaviour. Thus, it is based on behavioural principles of reward and punishment. In its application, reality orientation has been criticized for the punitive nature of some of its techniques. Furthermore, the validity of behavioural theory with people whose ability to change their behaviour is biologically impaired has been questioned. Nevertheless, some of the positive aspects of reality orientation – rewarding accurate memory rather than punishing confusion – can be usefully incorporated into direct work and assist families to minimize risk to confused relatives.

Validation therapy is not well known in Britain but has developed in America as an alternative method of working with confused people and is based on a set of different theoretical premises (Feil 1982). It may be applied to individual work or in groups but, like reality orientation, probably requires a degree of consistency which is difficult to achieve outside a residential or day setting. The method is based upon validation of the person and the primary aim is to understand 'the patient's view of reality in order to make meaningful emotional contact' (Feil 1991: 89). The approach is based upon three components: a theoretical view of development in older confused people; a four-fold categorization of the behaviour of confused people as they progress through the development of the illness; specific skills and methods of communication (verbal and non-verbal, including, where appropriate, touch) for people in each category. A crucial prerequisite to direct work is the assessment of the older person's behaviour in order to decide in which category or stage it best fits: malorientation, time confusion, repetitive motion or vegetation.

The method involves providing short periods of validation therapy each day – perhaps three sessions of five or ten minutes each for a maloriented person – with the aim of preventing the deterioration of behaviour into the next stage, and the skills can be developed by family members under the guidance of the worker. Skills are designed to encourage the older person to communicate, and this involves accepting the reality of the older person, but in a way which demonstrates respect and empathy and thus avoids infantilizing or demeaning the older person.

> For example: if the maloriented person says, 'I see a man under my bed,' the worker uses visual words to explore: 'What does the man look like? What is he wearing? Who does he remind you of? Is he tall?' If the maloriented person says, 'I hear voices at night', the validation worker builds trust by using hearing words: 'What does it sound like? Are the noises loud? Scratchy?' After 12 weeks of 5 minute validation sessions given three times per day, the validation worker asks: 'Is there a time when there is *no* man under your bed?' The . . . person may answer:

'When you are with me, he never comes. Maybe I don't want to be alone'.
(Feil 1991: 100–1)

The method has some strengths and its values are consistent with an anti-discriminatory approach. However, its effectiveness has not been evaluated extensively and few people in Britain have systematically applied it in practice.

Notwithstanding the criticisms discussed earlier about much of the practice of reminiscence groups (Harris and Hopkins 1994), which paradoxically have served to reinforce negative ageist stereotypes of older people, reminiscence and reminiscence groupwork can be applied in ways which both affirm confused older people and which therapeutically preserve or enhance cognitive, physical and social capacities. Gibson (1994: 47) distinguishes between general and specific reminiscence work which can be undertaken with individuals or groups:

> The term 'general' reminiscence work refers to well-prepared work that uses a variety of multi-sensory triggers to stimulate shared conversation on an agreed topic or those which relate loosely to the known background and interests of the participants. 'Specific' reminiscence work refers to carefully selected, highly-focused, concentrated consistent efforts to stimulate recall and conversation using carefully selected triggers known to closely approximate the detailed life-history of the participant.

Gibson's evaluation of a considerable number of reminiscence projects with confused older people suggests a number of possible benefits, although change is often small: reduction in agitation and restlessness, improved appetite, increased carer/staff understanding of individual older people. However, she stresses that this is skilled work for which group leaders and therapists need training. It must also be based upon explicit values which affirm older people and their personhood, and should not be implemented without systematic planning, briefing, debriefing, monitoring and evaluation based upon explicit objectives defined at the outset. The routine administration of organized reminiscence using standard equipment has no place in anti-ageist practice.

Death and dying: Grief and loss

It is not possible here to explore the vast literature upon these circumstances and the methods of working with people who are affected. Instead, there are two points which it is important for practitioners working with older people to understand. First, because old age is strongly associated with death, dying and loss (of other people and personal capacities), there may be a tendency for these issues to be taken less seriously when they affect older people. The assumption may be that because older people are closer to death and should therefore expect losses of various kinds, the impact when it occurs is less intense, less acute and less traumatic than with younger people. Thus, the loss of a partner of fifty years may be assumed to have less negative consequences than the loss of a partner of, say, ten or twenty years in middle age. Similarly, disability may be regarded as less of a crisis for an older than a younger person.

Such attitudes fail to account for the *subjective* meaning of loss for the older person and dehumanize the individual by the imposition of negative and discriminatory assumptions.

Second, and arising from the first point, is the view that, because these experiences are qualitatively different for older than younger people, older people faced with death or loss do not need the kind of interventions which younger people might expect, whether those interventions are concerned with grief counselling or the implementation of medical and other procedures to counter disabling conditions. The range of responses of older people to death, dying and loss are as wide as that among younger people, and this issue must be given sensitive, professional consideration by practitioners working with older people.

Sex and sexuality

One consequence of the loss of a partner is the loss of physical, intimate contact and sexual activity. Despite evidence that many older people continue to be sexually active, the myth persists that older men, and particularly older women, are uninterested in sex and, in any case, are usually incapable of engaging in sexual activity (Thienhaus *et al.* 1986). This is not to argue that all older people of all generations will be equally interested and active in sex. It is rather to argue that the assumption that sex generally plays little part in the lives of most older people is erroneous and ageist. The way in which people express themselves sexually will be in part determined by personal experience arising from characteristics such as age, gender, race as well as the social conventions prevailing when their attitudes to sex were shaped. Furthermore, attitudes change over time and the way we all behave sexually is moderated as circumstances, confidence and opportunity changes. Some people do undergo physical changes which can make sexual activity more uncomfortable, although assistance can be given, if the problem is acknowledged, in many cases. Similarly, the way in which sexual satisfaction is achieved can be adapted to accommodate disability.

The anti-discriminatory practitioner must recognize that issues of sex and sexuality may be very important to particular older people with whom they are working. Nevertheless, there are real dilemmas in raising these issues in ways which do not intrude inappropriately or affront the older person who regards such matters as absolutely private. It is possible to provide an opening for discussion, by furnishing the older person with the knowledge that the practitioner is sensitive to these issues, and by approaching the subject tangentially, through the generality of common experience rather than the specific circumstances of a particular individual. For example, talking to a women whose partner has died, the practitioner may say: 'One of the things other people often find they really miss is the physical contact and touching, especially in bed. Is that the same for you?'

Finally, it is also often assumed that, if older people have a sexual life, it must be heterosexual; gay and lesbian older people have experienced considerable difficulty in gaining social recognition and acceptance (Macdonald and Rich 1984). Same-sex cohabiters are assumed to be platonic friends and thereby experience strong barriers to disclosing the nature of their relationship. Practitioners must be able to entertain the possibility that, in later life, older people demonstrate a similar range and variety of personal, social and sexual relationships as younger people, while at the same time acknowledge the stereotypes which define them as asexual, post-sexual or, at best, strictly heterosexual beings.

Substance abuse

While most of the practice literature on substance abuse is focused upon young people, there has been some recognition that alcohol and other substances may be abused by a significant minority of older people. Substance abuse by older people, however, may be ignored or regarded as unimportant because of an attitude that the damage it causes is less significant for a person nearer the end of life (Scrutton 1989). However, not only may alcohol, for example, be more damaging to organs in older bodies, abusive consumption may be due to problems of living with which the older person needs help. The approach to substance abuse is essentially that adopted with younger people: a balance of rights and risks; informed discussion of the reasons for and consequences of continued abuse; counselling; strategies to reduce or curtail consumption if the older person agrees. Once again the main issues for practitioners are (1) to be able to recognize substance abuse in older people and (2) to apply the same knowledge and skills developed for working with other abusers, with a focus upon the older person as an adult whose consent to participation in a withdrawal programme is essential.

8

Protection

The question whether older people are abused and, if so, to what extent and in what circumstances has gathered momentum over recent years, although in Britain uncertainty prevails about the most likely answers. During the late 1970s and 1980s, American gerontologists and sociologists began to examine systematically the 'battered elder syndrome', an early term which resonated with the disparaging 'granny-battering' label which first emerged in Britain (Baker 1975). Such terminology arguably reflected the ambivalence with which the seriousness and significance of the phenomenon was then regarded. However, as research in the USA and Canada (followed by studies in Britain) began to chart the incidence, prevalence and nature of mistreatment of older people, and as the issue of care of older people became more politicized, particularly in the USA, these terms were superseded by others which acknowledged the gravity of the issue – elder abuse and neglect, old age abuse, elder mistreatment.

However, agreement about acceptable terminology is about the limit of consensus so far, apart from a general acceptance that older people are abused and that the extent of reported abuse probably underestimates the incidence to a significant degree. Partly because our understanding and mapping of elder abuse is in its infancy and partly because early studies did not use common definitions or methods upon which a body of knowledge could be built, there remains considerable uncertainty about definitions, incidence, prevalence and the factors associated with abuse (Decalmer and Glendenning 1993). Consequently, professionals have been slow to recognize abuse, and practice in individual cases has been characterized by delay and uncertainty in intervention and a lack of procedural guidelines within agencies (SSI 1992). The absence of any clear legal basis for intervention reflects the fact that, so far, government has rejected the need for legislation to protect vulnerable adults.

This chapter will examine (1) current thinking in relation to definitions, (2) the incidence, prevalence and characteristics of abuse, and (3) theoretical explanations of abuse and neglect. I then propose a conceptual framework for understanding elder abuse and, finally, I consider the factors associated with the risk of abuse and the task facing professional helpers, particularly in relation to assessment and intervention.

What is elder abuse?

A plethora of definitions, each developed into a particular typology of abuse, has made it more difficult to develop a definitional consensus around which progress may be made. In part, this situation has arisen because different 'investigators have approached elder abuse from different perspectives: the victim, the carer, the physician, the nurse, the agency, the social worker, social policy; and, as a result, there has been a lack of clarity' (Glendenning 1993: 5). A further complication is that, while some commentators have sought to develop typologies or categories of abuse, others have focused upon conceptualization, attempting to articulate a more fundamental theoretical explanation and way of understanding the characteristics of the abuse which research was beginning to reveal. Thus, in defining, describing and conceptualizing abuse of older people, a number of key issues remain unresolved. For example, should neglect be included in a definition of elder abuse? Should active neglect be distinguished from passive neglect? Is self-neglect abusive? Is exploitation by others abusive? Should sexual abuse be considered as a variant of physical abuse or is it inherently different and therefore a separate category? When does verbal aggression become psychologically abusive? And, even more fundamentally, is elder abuse a distinct social phenomenon or is it a previously unrecognized form of intra-family violence (Bennett and Kingston 1993)?

Definitions

Most definitions emphasize the carer/cared-for relationship as the context of abuse and thereby focus immediately on the level of interpersonal relationships as the primary factor. One of the first definitions of elder abuse to appear in Britain also located abuse within the carer/cared-for relationship (Eastman 1984). While Eastman identified power and power differentials within relationships as the core issues, in other respects it is limited. The implied context of abuse is that of *individual* dependency and interpersonal relationships based on caring. As such, the definition takes no account of the *structured* dependency of older people as a group, nor of current and past relationships which are not constructed upon care but which rather reflect historical roles, changes in role or previous patterns of interpersonal behaviour. There has been considerable debate about whether 'intentionality' on the part of the perpetrator should be an essential characteristic of abuse. However, as Riley (1989) pointed out, definitions should concentrate on the effect on the abused elder, who is as much at risk whether the abuse is deliberate or not. Thus, it is generally accepted that acts of omission as well as commission constitute abuse. However, there remains uncertainty as to whether self-neglect or self-harm should be defined as abusive.

The lack of clarity about definitions reflects in part a struggle not only with language and semantics but also conceptualization. One difficulty is the label 'abuse', which implies intentionality and deliberation. If the exploration of elder mistreatment had started from the perspective of considering *risk* to older people, the inclusion of self-neglect, passive or unintentional neglect by others, exploitation as well as risk of poverty and marginalization arising from macro-level policies would not be so problematic. However, the labelling of older people 'at risk' runs counter to the trends within theory and practice to empower older people and to challenge negative, ageist stereotypes of older people as inherently vulnerable and dependent. The 'definitional disarray' identified by Pillemer and Finkelhor in 1988 is yet to be significantly improved.

Typologies

While a consensus about definitions has not been reached, there is a core of agreement that elder abuse exists, it is under-reported, and that it includes physical assaults, psychological harassment, neglect and exploitation. Glendenning (1993) has produced a comprehensive summary of the different typologies developed by researchers and practitioners over the last fifteen years. More recently, local authorities and some health authorities have published typologies in procedural guides and policy statements and there have been some developments at the national level aimed at developing a more systematic approach to the definition of abuse and professional responses to it (SSI 1993).

The typology in Table 8.1 is the result of an analysis of typologies proposed within key texts and represents a comprehensive list of types of abuse about which there is a degree of consensus among at least some, if not all, of the main commentators. In producing this typology, however, I have also made some particular decisions with which not everyone may agree. For example, sexual abuse is included as a separate category rather than as a type of physical abuse because it involves the transgression of quite distinct social taboos and is probably characterized, as with other forms of sexual abuse, by a distinct gender pattern between victim and abuser which may not characterize physical violence. The typology also incorporates abuse which arises not only from behaviour between individuals but also from legitimized and officially or unofficially sanctioned routine practices within institutions. The issue of institutionalized abuse will be discussed more fully in a later section.

Particular acts may not fit neatly into one or other category. For example, sexual abuse may also involve a degree of physical violence. Physical assault over a period of time will undoubtedly generate psychological fear. Locking an elderly person in a room for a prolonged period results in physical isolation and psychological distress. The routine administration of sedatives at bedtime in a residential home is institutionalized abuse which physically assaults the residents to whom it is given unnecessarily. Failure to inform residents of their right to vote is an institutionalized practice which constitutes a violation of individual rights. Policies which deny medical treatment, usually for acute

Table 8.1 Typology of elder abuse and neglect

Physical abuse	Physical assault, violence; restriction of movement by physical means; unjustified restraint; burning; sedation; misuse or maladministration of drugs; sleep deprivation
Sexual abuse	Sexual activity which the older person does not freely and meaningfully consent to; inappropriate touching of the breasts, genitals, etc.
Psychological abuse	Verbal aggression; provoking fear or distress through words or actions; harassment; ridicule; name-calling; threatening behaviour; forced isolation
Material abuse	Appropriation of money or material effects; misrepresentation; theft; gaining consent to finance/financial control through devious or unethical means
Neglect	Withholding of necessary physical care; malnourishment; maintaining older person in dirty conditions; failure to toilet; withholding of food
Violation of rights	Actions which limit or deny human or civil rights to elderly persons within their community, residential institution or family
Self-abuse	Physical abuse, neglect or violation of rights by the older person him or herself
Institutionalized abuse	Abuse, neglect or violation of rights of an older person or persons which results from routinized and officially or unofficially sanctioned practices at the level of management or care practice within a hospital, group care or residential institution

conditions, to persons above a certain age are institutionalized policies which violate civil and human rights. Furthermore, a typology will not necessarily assist in those situations in which practices which could be described as abusive appear to be necessary for the protection of older people whose mental facilities are limited. For example, if a relative keeps doors in the home locked because otherwise a confused older person would wander, should this be classed as abusive? There is a clear argument that, in this context, such practice is not abusive, even though it would be judged so if the older person were mentally lucid and the locked doors used to restrain her. Thus, a typology will not resolve the dilemmas which arise in practice, nor will it obviate the need for systematic assessment which takes account of the actual behaviours, the characteristics of the people involved and the context within which they are living.

Prevalence, incidence and characteristics of abuse

Reported rates of prevalence (the number of cases of abuse within the population) and incidence (the number of new cases appearing within, say, a year) vary widely and, moreover, the rates reported in different studies are not comparable, based as they are on different definitions, sampling techniques and research methods. The vast majority of studies are also based on cases of abuse known to the helping agencies of one kind or another. Furthermore, many estimates of abuse in Britain have been calculated by applying prevalence rates derived from American studies to British population figures, a technique of uncertain validity (e.g. Eastman 1984; Ogg and Bennett 1992). Nevertheless, the rates of elder abuse in British households derived from these studies have varied from an estimated 500,000 people 'at risk' (Eastman 1984); 10 per cent at risk and 1 in 1000 actually suffering physical abuse (Hocking 1988); and 8 out of a patient register of 200 suffering abuse or inadequate care (Ogg and Bennett 1992).

The most significant study, based on a large random-sample survey of 2000 older people in Boston, USA, reported a prevalence rate of 32 per 1000, with physical violence the most commonly reported ($n = 20$), followed by verbal aggression ($n = 11$) and neglect ($n = 4$) (Pillemer and Finkelhor 1988). The results of this study are likely to be more reliable because of the large sample size, its random selection and, in particular, because the sample was drawn from the general population of older people rather than from a register of patients or agency referrals. Even so, it is likely that specific types of abuse were under-reported, particularly sexual and material abuse, and it did not include people resident in residential or nursing homes. While Pillemer and Finkelhor have provided the most reliable figures to date, they paint only a partial picture, from which we can only conclude that elder abuse is not less and is likely to be more than the rates reported in this study.

Research into cases of alleged or known abuse have also examined the characteristics of victims and abusers. Once again, these studies are limited in that their findings are based on the relatively small proportion of cases that are reported and thus may present a distorted picture. Furthermore, the collation of characteristics of individual cases inevitably focuses upon the micro-context of familial life and personal attributes and thus fails to locate the findings within the wider context of prevailing social policy and attitudes. On the basis of these studies, it was suggested that victims were more likely to be very old, white women, aged 80 years or more, with dementia, physical disability or cerebrovascular disease (Hocking 1988). Older people who have difficulty in communicating or experience fluctuating disability were also shown to be at higher risk. In reported cases, abusers tend to be an adult child in the principal carer role, frequently a victim themselves of sickness or isolation, with a higher than expected history of alcohol or drug abuse, mental illness, unemployment, and a history of a poor relationship with the elderly person (Cloke 1983; Homer and Gilleard 1990; McCreadie 1991). Thus, the picture which emerges from studies of known or suspected cases portrays a stressed or pathological abuser in the role of carer of a burdensome, dependent, very old woman, almost always white. Cases provided by a range of health and social services workers in London for a study by the Department of Health (SSI 1992) echoed these findings and prompted the authors to note, in the light of the population from which the cases were drawn:

> . . . it would seem reasonable to expect more evidence of abuse among ethnic elders . . . and it therefore seems possible that this section of the population was overlooked when cases were being selected: in any case, it

seems likely that the needs of ethnic elders in relation to elder abuse have not been recognised.

(SSI 1992: 415)

Pillemer and Finkelhor's (1988) study also produced findings which challenge the prevailing stereotype of elder abuse. In their random sample of elderly people living in the community, more elderly men than women reported abuse and, of the perpetrators, a majority (58 per cent) were spouses and only 24 per cent were adult children. In other respects, the study confirmed earlier findings: abused elderly people were more likely to be living with another person, to be economically or materially disadvantaged and, if neglected, to be isolated and have little support. However, the emphasis upon abuse within a marital relationship and of a much greater proportion of male victims than previously supposed was a considerable challenge to previous assumptions and led the authors to call for future studies of elder abuse to be based upon general population surveys. However, the ethical and methodo-logical difficulties posed by such research are not easily surmountable (Ogg and Munn-Giddings 1993).

The message for practitioners is clear. We tend to recognize elder abuse only when it occurs in situations which conform to our expectations: elder abuse happens when an adult child is over-burdened with the care of a very old female relative whose faculties and abilities for self-care have significantly deteriorated. This is also the kind of domestic situation most likely to come to the attention of a service agency. However, the research suggests that abuse is more likely to occur in other kinds of domestic arrangements, notably between spouses, and therefore at the very least practitioners should have a more open and questioning approach to the possibility of elder abuse in a wider range of circumstances.

Theoretical explanations of elder abuse

Most of the literature focuses upon explaining abuse and neglect at the level of victim–abuser interaction. Phillips (1986) identified three theoretical ap-proaches which had emerged from the empirical data: the situational model, exchange theory and symbolic interactionism. Biggs and Phillipson (1992) also add to this list the social construction of old age, which will be used in the next section to develop an alternative model for conceptualizing elder abuse.

The situational model

This perspective identifies the stress within a situation as the key factor which precipitates abuse. Stress may be derived from a number of different sources: the *abuser* may have a low stress threshold because of his or her personal characteristics, drug/alcohol dependency, previous experiences of violence, previous relationship with the elder person; the *elderly person* may add to a high stress level in the situation through high dependency, impaired mental health, personality factors; *structural* factors such as poverty, isolation, poor environ-mental amenities may contribute to stress overload. However, while this perspective appears to be the one most readily adopted by practitioners, Phillips found that the data available did not fit readily with the model, mainly because of the difficulty in comparing studies with different definitions and methods. She concluded that the situational model may not be appropriate.

Exchange theory

This perspective focuses upon the reciprocity, or social exchange, which is characteristic of mutually satisfying relationships. Relationships are conceptualized as systems of rewards and punishments, in which partners seek to maximize the rewards, or benefits, for each other. A failure to achieve an overall balance of mutual rewards may result in conflict and, consequently, abuse. In family situations involving older people, it is argued, the potential for an imbalance of mutual rewards may arise if the older person is more vulnerable, more dependent and less able to contribute in a positive way to the relationship. However, this assumption leads to the conclusion that abuse is more likely when the older person is more dependent, whereas 'researchers have failed to produce unequivocal evidence that abused elders are more dependent than non-abused elders' (Glendenning 1993: 25).

Symbolic interactionism

While symbolic interactionism also focuses upon relationships as the key context within which abuse has to be understood, it signals the importance for family members of the *meaning* of their relationships and argues that the roles which people adopt towards one another have to be constantly negotiated and renegotiated throughout the life course. As people age or change, they have to reach a new consensus with significant others as to the new roles and relationships which will exist between them. Unless such consensus is reached, conflict or termination of the relationship will ensue. Elder abuse, within this model, can arise when either the older person cannot fulfil a meaningful role *vis-à-vis* the other person, or when a consensus about changed roles cannot be achieved; for example, in the case of an elderly mother changing from 'carer/parent' to 'cared-for' individual, or an independent adult child accepting caring responsibilities. This perspective explains abuse in terms of the conflict that can arise when identities and roles change and a new contract cannot be agreed.

All three models described above focus upon interpersonal relationships and identify the catalyst for abuse as the breakdown or stress within those relationships. To a greater or lesser extent, they each identify causative factors within the older person: dependency; inability to reciprocate; failure to execute a meaningful role. As such, they are in danger of persecuting the victim: making the older person in some way responsible for the abuse to which they are subjected.

This is not to argue that some older people do not provoke anger or violence, or are difficult and demanding to care for. This is true of individuals from all groups in society who experience abuse: children, women, black people, disabled people. However, while it may be recognized that, in individual instances, the behaviour of the victim may contribute to the emotional level of a situation which then becomes abusive, this understanding at the level of the individual has not been elevated to the scale of a general theory through which abuse of other groups of people, say children, can be understood. The difference in relation to elder abuse is that the stereotypical characteristics of older people *as a group* and perceived characteristics of old age have been used as a causatory factor in explaining the abuse and, by so doing, the victim–abuser relationship has been subverted. The victim has become the persecutor; the abuser is the victim of stress or unrewarding, demanding relationships.

Theories to explain other forms of family violence, such as child abuse or domestic violence against women, look beyond the microcosm of individual interpersonal dynamics to power inequalities, social attitudes and economic discrimination as essential factors in the wider societal context within which such abuse has to be understood. It is an indication of the deep-rootedness of ageism and its pervasion throughout all aspects of political and social life that elderly people have been made responsible, at least in part, for their own abuse.

A conceptual framework for understanding elder abuse

Abuse between two people can occur only if a power imbalance exists between them: one person believes himself, and is perceived by the other, to be more powerful; the other believes himself, and is perceived, to be relatively powerless. The belief and the perception are not necessarily conscious; they are derived through the minutiae of interactions which take place in daily life and the establishment of patterns of interaction which confirm and reinforce the relative positions of one as more powerful and the other as less powerful.

The establishment of relative positions of power, however, is not solely derived from the idiosyncratic characteristics of personal qualities, personal histories and interpersonal dynamics. The characteristics imbued in individuals by their membership of particular groups in society give some people the inherent advantage of more power, whereas others are relatively disadvantaged in the power stakes because they are members of groups whose structural position in society is weaker.

This is a complex argument and one which may be difficult to grasp, since it is concerned with the interface between the personal and the political: the way in which the power structures of society infiltrate, to a greater or lesser extent, our personal lives and, indeed, intimate relationships. Perhaps gender relationships are the most straightforward example of this process. Politically, economically and socially, men are more powerful than women and this is evidenced in every facet of social life as men are disproportionately represented in the highest echelons of power. Despite women making up more than half the population, they are relatively powerless. This structural inequality is not natural or inevitable; it is produced, sustained, reinforced and continually reproduced by social conventions, attitudes, differential opportunities and expectations of women and men, manufactured through the differential socialization of girls and boys. These structures are not immutable but are very difficult to change. It is hardly surprising that many men and women internalize, to some degree, the conventional wisdom as to their relative power *vis-à-vis* one another. Without a perception that men are more powerful, rape and domestic violence against women could not occur on the scale it does. The factors which trigger individual instances of violence are important but secondary: the context of a perception of power inequality in the home buttressed by power inequality in society is the primary context which allows such violence to occur.

A similar analysis has to be applied to the understanding of elder abuse and the starting point must be the social construction of ageing within Western societies, the politically and economically weak position of older people, the structured dependency enforced upon older people as a group and the negative stereotypes of old age which support and justify their structural inequality. Chapters 2 and 3 have developed this theoretical analysis, and it will not be repeated here. However, the consequence of the structured dependency of older people and negative stereotypes of old age at the level of personal life is the view that older people are relatively less powerful, and it is this perceived power differential which allows abuse of older people to occur.

To this extent, elder abuse shares a common basis with other forms of familial and interpersonal violence and the development of a theoretical framework must begin with a similar analysis of interpersonal power differentials and their origins in wider social structures. However, building upon this fundamental analysis, a theoretical framework of elder abuse will at some point diverge from those developed to explain child abuse or domestic violence. Abuse of elders shares some important commonalities with other forms of abuse, but it is also characterized by some important differences which must be accounted for. For example, older people are adults, not children, and therefore it would be inappropriate to draw too many parallels between child and elder abuse. On the other hand, many elderly people are physically or mentally frail to a degree which most abused adult women are not. Furthermore, the relationships of child/parent, woman/male partner, elderly person/spouse, elder/adult child embody quite fundamental differences which must be understood at the interpersonal level. Thus, a conceptual framework for understanding elder abuse must:

- begin from an analysis of the context of ageism and old age inequality;
- connect conceptually different forms of abuse at different levels in society;
- locate domestic and institutional abuse of individual older people within the wider context of social attitudes;
- offer an explanation for current levels and types of abuse;
- offer an explanation why not all elderly people are abused;
- suggest factors, within the overall analysis, which might predict abusive and non-abusive situations.

Figure 8.1 represents schematically a conceptual framework for elder abuse which is based upon an analysis of the power inequality of older people embedded in social structures and attitudes and which illustrates the inextricable interconnectedness of political and personal levels of experience. It also attempts to demonstrate how abuse of individual older people must be understood as a variant of other legitimized forms of abuse within institutional practice and state policies:

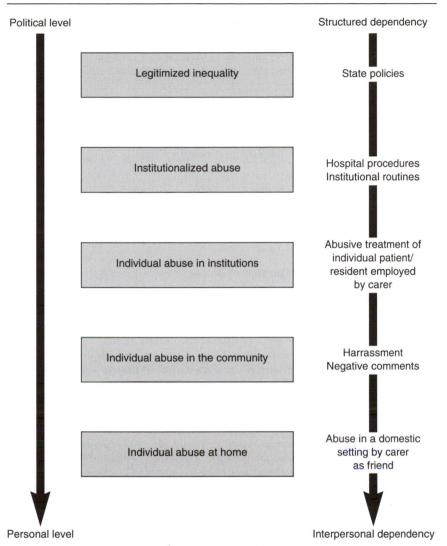

Political level   Structured dependency

Legitimized inequality   State policies

Institutionalized abuse   Hospital procedures
                                                   Institutional routines

Individual abuse in institutions   Abusive treatment of
                                                   individual patient/
                                                   resident employed
                                                   by carer

Individual abuse in the community   Harrassment
                                                   Negative comments

Individual abuse at home   Abuse in a domestic
                                                   setting by carer
                                                   as friend

Personal level   Interpersonal dependency

Figure 8.1   Ageism and elder abuse: a conceptual framework

1 *Legitimized inequality.* State policies frequently discriminate in negative ways
   against older people. Chapter 2 illustrated how the income maintenance
   system denies disabled older people benefits afforded to younger disabled
   people. Older people receive less income, as a group, and experience poorer
   housing and material circumstances.
2 *Institutionalized abuse.* Institutionalized abuse is the routine depersonaliz-
   ation of, or discrimination against, groups of older people in particular
   settings. The implementation of procedures in many institutions abuses
   older people. For example, many hospitals are said to have official or

unofficial policies which deny intensive care to people over 65 or 70 years admitted with heart attacks; residential and nursing homes have been shown to have routinized practices or inadequate care procedures which result in abuse. Several enquiries have identified abuse through routine practices.

3 *Individual abuse in institutions.* In addition to institutionalized abuse in hospitals and care establishments, individual older people have been targeted for abuse by particular nursing or care staff. Institutions, because of their semi-closed environment and the intimate nature of the care required, appear to be environments in which abuse can occur unreported for significant periods of time.

4 *Individual abuse in the community.* Hostile attitudes, negative comments, disparaging remarks, harrassment by employees in shops, on buses.

5 *Individual abuse at home.* Abuse of older people by a relative, friend, neighbour or paid carer in their own home or a relative's domestic environment.

Factors associated with the risk of abuse

Having located the abuse of individual older people within the context of ageist attitudes and values, there remains the question as to why some older people are abused and others are not. Indeed, the question could be reformulated as follows: 'Why are not more older people abused?' The answer to this question is two-fold. First, it is likely that significantly more older people *are* abused than the evidence suggests, and within the conceptual framework developed this would be predictable. Second, the framework defines a context within which abuse, while not permissible, becomes possible. It does not predict that all elderly people *will* be abused. It is clear that many relationships are based on factors other than power differentials. Indeed, in some families, older people *are* afforded power and status by virtue of family values which transcend social values or because of the history of positive relationships which have developed over many years. Whether abuse occurs in an individual situation will depend on a balance of other factors, some of which will tend to increase the power inequality and therefore tend to increase the risk of abuse, others which will counterbalance or reduce the power inequality and so decrease the risk of abuse.

Using case analysis, several studies have identified the factors which appear to be associated with a high risk of abuse, although their significance in relation to power inequalities has not been analysed (O'Malley *et al.* 1979; Breckman and Adelman 1988). Breckman and Adelman (1988) have identified six key risk factors associated with abuse:

1 *Psychopathology on the part of the abuser.* This may be a history of mental illness, substance abuse or violent behaviour, factors which may suggest a personality or personal experience which reduces the ability of the abuser to refrain from abusing a position of relative power.

2 *Trans-generational violence.* If the family has developed a pattern of abusing power and using violence as a means of demonstrating power over others, then this pattern is also more likely to be repeated with elderly members.

3 *Dependency*. A high level of physical or mental dependency increases still further the power imbalance between the elderly person and others and may increase the differential so far that the abuser is tipped towards behaviour patterns normally reserved for extremely powerless people (i.e. children). Alternatively, dependency in other family members may reduce the abuser's tolerance of dependency in the older adult.

4 *Stress*. Stress can produce uncharacteristic behaviour patterns in many human situations and, when one adult is more powerful, abuse may result.

5 *Isolation*. Isolation from other people can also produce uncharacteristic behaviour: everyone needs the checks and balances that contact with others brings. We moderate our own behaviour in accordance with the expectations of others and refrain from deviant behaviour partly because we are observed. Isolated people not only experience greater stress through lack of social contact, but may also lose the inhibitions which contact imposes.

6 *Living arrangements*. Sharing accommodation with another person increases the opportunity for abuse, as well as contributing to stress in certain families.

O'Malley and co-workers' (1979) early study identified a number of conditions associated with the risk of abuse: severe cognitive impairment; severe physical impairment; depression; talk of punishment by elder or carer; a family norm of violence; isolation; refusal of services; control of elder's finances; inconsistency of information. This is rather a mixed list, including both factors associated with risk of abuse and indicators that abuse may be taking place. A study by Pillemer (1986), comparing abusive and non-abusive matched cases, identified five factors similar to those of Breckman and Adelman: intra-individual dynamics (psychopathology of the abuser); inter-generational transmission (cycle of violence); dependency and exchange relationships between abused and abuser; external stress; social isolation.

Signs of abuse

A number of studies have identified a wide range of indicators which may suggest that abuse is taking place. However, as with all indicators, their status is suggestive and not predictive. Each of these indicators could be explained by a different, non-abusive condition and therefore they must be applied cautiously as an *aid* to assessment and not used alone to diagnose abuse. The indicators may be grouped into those which describe the abused person and those which describe the abuser.

Abused person recurring or unexplained injuries,
failure to treat medical conditions,
poor hygiene,
lack of adequate nourishment,
dehydration,
unexplained bruises,
depression,
withdrawal or tearfulness,
imposed restraint or isolation,
lack of comfort relative to means,

unexplained genital/urinary infections,
soiled bedlinen or clothing,
unexplained/unexpected deterioration in health,
absence of necessary aids such as spectacles or dentures,
over-sedation, misuse of medication,
unexplained changes in behaviour or routine,
denial of abuse or problems.

Abuser   denial of medical treatment to elder,
refusal of services,
failure to keep appointments,
erratic behaviour,
inconsistent information or accounts of injuries,
volatile behaviour/verbal aggression,
behaviour indicating stress,
denial of rights and authority to elder,
control of assets and decision-making.

The above lists were compiled with reference to Glendenning (1993) and Breckman and Adelman (1988).

The professional task

Issues and dilemmas

While a number of local authorities have followed the lead of central government departments (ADSS 1991; SSI 1993) and developed policy and procedural guidelines for elder abuse, there is still a lack of knowledge and practice wisdom at the local level. Indeed, some of the guidelines are already outdated, relying heavily on partial knowledge and infused with an uncritical acceptance of 'carer strain theory' as the underlying explanation for most abuse. As Penhale (1993: 109) has noted:

> . . . existing guidelines available concerning the identification of (and intervention in) situations of elder abuse do not match the complexities of the cases which professionals are working with and the knowledge base is actually quite limited.

The hegemony of 'carer strain theory' is exemplified in the guidelines of one local authority, whose discussion of the role of the professional in cases of elder abuse argues: '. . . when an unpaid carer constantly copes with an elderly relative whose behaviour is highly challenging, and eventually breaks down under this pressure, there may be real doubts about who is abusing whom' (Rochdale SSD 1993: 7). This statement is arguably a subversion of the principles upon which the professional task should be based, and reflects the discriminatory attitudes to elder victims which would not be tolerated in relation to women or child victims.

Professionals, then, face a number of difficult dilemmas working in an arena in which the development of good practice is in its infancy (Riley 1989). It is important, therefore, that the professional task is based upon some key principles:

- *Awareness*: practitioners must not only have an accurate and extensive knowledge of elder abuse, but be sufficiently aware to recognize abusive or potentially abusive situations. Otherwise, elder abuse will continue to pass unnoticed.
- *Acceptance*: it is important that the values underpinning practice include an acceptance that elder abuse occurs and that it *is* abuse. This involves a conscious attempt to avoid the insidious slide into 'carer strain theory' and to adopt a neutral stance at the point of investigation, assessment and intervention.
- *Good practice*: the professional response to suspected elder abuse should be based upon a systematic process of investigation, assessment, intervention and care management which incorporates the use of relevant legislation; the collation of relevant information; liaison with the police; the use of the case conference; a clear relationship between the type of abuse, assessed causes and methods of intervention (Pritchard 1992: 163).

The professional task in most cases is likely to be extremely complex and the professional route through the situation is often obscured by a number of features that are common in elder abuse:

- *Victim reluctance*. For a variety of reasons, including fear of the consequences, reluctance to name a relative, and dependence upon the abuser, victims may be reluctant to disclose, or even admit to themselves, that abuse is taking place. However, adult victims have the right to refuse services. Professionals will be faced with a difficult task of balancing issues of protection on the one hand and rights to self-determination on the other.
- *Abuser resistance*. Denial is also a likely first response of many abusers, unable to predict the consequences or to face the perceived stigma of an admission.
- *Practitioner powerlessness*. Many practitioners may feel powerless in the face of suspected elder abuse, not only in response to the complex dynamics of a particular case, but also because of the professional context which includes no specific legislative basis and probably only a limited number of options for intervention, particularly if the abuser is a carer and intervention is likely to result in a need for different care arrangements.
- *Situational isolation*. In many cases, elders are not routinely connected to other situations in which abuse may become visible, or from which further information during an investigation may help with the assessment process. Older people, unlike other victims, are not employed or in full-time education and many are unlikely to be connected with a particular situation outside the home with sufficient regularity or frequency for injuries or changes in appearance or behaviour to be noticed. Furthermore, in cases which are abusive, isolation is likely to be extreme.

Investigation, assessment and intervention

In general, the principles and process of a comprehensive multidisciplinary assessment should be adopted and Chapter 5 has described in detail a particular model which could be used. National guidelines have endorsed the view that, in cases of suspended elder abuse, assessment should be 'needs-led and holistic' and concerned with the degree of dependency and disability, as well as risk and stress factors, assessed within a multi-agency approach (SSI 1993). The time needed for assessment will vary and should not be limited to a single visit (Francis 1993). All guidelines agree that the older person should be interviewed alone if possible and certainly not in the presence of a suspected abuser.

Consideration should be given to the calling of a case conference and careful planning should be undertaken to determine who, including the older person and carer, should attend and for which parts of the meeting. As with all case conferences, detailed preparation is essential and the knowledge and skills of the chairperson are crucial to both the process and outcome of the decision-making. The assessment formulated for the case conference should include all the elements of a comprehensive multidisciplinary assessment, with the addition of a detailed description of the incident or allegations and the responses of key individuals, including the victim and suspected abuser(s).

The case conference should assess the facts in the light of available knowledge of elder abuse and should form a judgement about the likelihood that abuse has taken place. It needs to assess:

- the type and probable causes of the abuse;
- the risk of further abuse;
- immediate action including use of legislation;
- objectives for the immediate future;
- identification of the key worker/care manager;
- arrangements and time-scale for review.

The objectives of intervention must be related clearly to the analysis of type and causes of abuse. Research has indicated that when abuse is identified or alleged, the most common action is the organization of some kind of support services, without any indication of their relevance for reducing the risk of further abuse. The care manager must address the assessed risk and aim to provide a package of care or services which eliminates or reduces risk. The provison of support in the vague hope it will achieve this aim is not an adequate professional response.

9

Conclusion: Challenges and priorities

Introduction

> As the Act, its antecedent White Paper and its later guidance and implementation documents make plain, health and social care decision-making will be bottom-up, needs-led, and multi-agency, with innovations encouraged by financial and other incentives and system implications couched in terms of social and not merely public expenditures.
>
> (Malin 1994: 4, commenting upon Knapp *et al.* 1993)

> It seems a faint hope that an administrative model which may involve setting unattainable standards based on competence-led performance indicators, inflexibility in eligibility criteria, and limitations on the use of self as a resource, can supply the incentives to provide or even to broker services in an improved way. To propose that separation of assessment from provision might provide a better incentive to create a needs-led service, than professional judgement, is to show a degree of confusion about the origins of our present predicament (shortage of resource; bureaucratisation, etc.) bordering on the incredible.
>
> (Huxley 1993: 378)

Knapp and Huxley illustrate the extent to which opinions diverge as to whether the community care legislation and its associated administrative arrangements will lead to improved outcomes for users and carers, particularly in terms of the key criteria of choice, quality, participation and empowerment. The crucial issues revolve not so much around the processes of assessment and care management *per se*, but the welfare market and contract culture with which community care has been imprinted. The Introduction to the book identified the potential for contradiction and tension between the service objectives and the wider political objectives entwined within the legislation and its subsequent guidance. On the one hand, service objectives emphasize user choice, flexibility and participation within a wide range of domiciliary services. Political imperatives, on the other hand, require local authorities to create internal and external markets and to redefine significantly their role *vis-à-vis* users and carers. This chapter first identifies two aspects of the community care arrangements which present specific challenges to the development of anti-discriminatory, user/carer-oriented practice. Second, the chapter and the book conclude with an agenda of priorities to which practitioners and managers can subscribe in their attempts to minimize the challenges and maximize the potential to deliver high-quality, anti-discriminatory community care to older people and carers.

Challenges

The market system and the new managerial approach with which it is associated inevitably tends towards an *administrative model of community care*, in which assessment and care management are processes designed primarily to support managerial objectives and resource allocation priorities. Table 9.1 describes the essential elements of an administrative model of community care: an organizationally oriented system aimed at rationing scarce resources and intervening at the lowest level possible. This is a model which reduces the scope for professional judgement to a minimum and defines care management as a technical task, a 'pick and mix' exercise, matching available services to needs which are largely defined in straightforward, practical ways. The

Table 9.1　Models of community care: The administrative model

Focus	*Organizationally oriented*	A model designed primarily to ration resources according to organizationally defined criteria
Assessment	*Managerial*	Assessment as the vehicle for managing and justifying how resources are allocated
Care management	*Administrative*	Designed to fit resources to defined needs in accordance with a specified budget. Care manager as administrator
Definition of need	*Limited*	The system is designed to define need as that requiring the lowest level of intervention
Content	*Practical*	Assessment and care management emphasize needs which can be met through practical services
Scope	*Reductional*	The system is designed to reduce both the concept of need *and* the complexity of the issues facing the user and carer
Skills	*Technical*	Emphasizes skills of organizing managing and administrating
Definition of outcome	*Service deficits*	The effectiveness of the system is defined as unmet needs and the services required to meet them

effectiveness of the system is defined in administrative terms with outcome measured in terms of service deficits rather than user satisfaction. Lewis (1994) has argued that the tendency towards an administrative model would be greater in a context of limited resources.

A second challenge arises from a consequence of the introduction of a market system into the organization and delivery of welfare: the redesignation of practitioners as either *purchasers or providers* and the separation of these two functions at different levels with the organization. While senior management, with their strategic planning role, clearly must have a commissioning function, many agencies have also introduced a purchaser–provider split at the managerial and operational levels. Thus, middle managers, team leaders and front-line practitioners are increasingly being located either within a purchasing division or a providing division, with consequent implications for their role, task and function. The potential to retain a holistic professional approach in which assessment, professional judgement and a wide range of professional skills are integrated within the user–practitioner relationship is seriously challenged by these organizational arrangements. Indeed, some commentators have questioned the extent to which such a split is both conceptually and practically feasible in the day-to-day relationships practitioners have with older people and their carers (Huxley 1993).

Voluntary organizations, in particular, have been adversely affected by the separation of purchaser and provider roles. In many areas, voluntary organizations have been excluded from the strategic commissioning level on the grounds that, as potential providers of services in a contract relationship with the local authority, there is an inherent conflict of interest which properly excludes them from decisions concerned with service planning and strategic commissioning. However, voluntary organizations have arguably also regarded themselves, perhaps primarily, as commentators upon the needs of service users and as agitators for better services, with a claim to be able to speak with and for users in a special way. This voice is now being excluded from the strategic planning process, the key players of which are increasingly represented solely by the statutory local authority and health sectors.

The tendency towards an administrative model of community care, and the organizational separation of purchasing (assessment) and providing, together constitute a significant challenge not only to the development of an anti-discriminatory approach but also to the user-oriented objectives of the legislation itself. The reductionist values inherent in these changes are not consistent with the need for a structure and process which can accommodate complexity, see older people as a highly differentiated group with diverse needs and characteristics, and demand of practitioners the integrated holistic skills essential for the provision of a high-quality, coordinated service to the user and carer.

Priorities

There are a number of key priorities which practitioners can adopt as part of a professional agenda to minimize the consequences of these challenges and

Table 9.2   Models of community care: The professional model

Focus	User/carer-oriented	A model designed to start from and integrate fully the user/carer perspective and participation
Assessment	*Professional*	Assessment as the process for establishing a holistic picture of needs
Care management	*Therapeutic*	Designed to engage user/carer in fitting resources to needs. Care manager also addresses therapeutic needs through the process
Definition of needs	*Extended*	The system is designed to explore and elaborate a wide range of needs and develop a holistic view
Content	*Practical and emotional*	Assessment and care management emphasize needs and experiences which require both practical and therapeutic help
Scope	*Elaborative*	The system is designed to incorporate a holistic definition of need, an understanding of the complexity of issues facing the user/carer, and a perspective which acknowledges diversity and life history
Skills	*Complex*	Emphasizes the equal importance of interpersonal, therapeutic and administrative skills
Definition of outcome	*Client satisfaction and outcome*	The effectiveness of the system is defined in terms of outcomes for people: satisfaction, improvement in their situation, unmet need

enhance the possibility of preserving and developing high-quality, anti-discriminatory practice with older people and their carers.

1 *The professional model.* Practitioners and managers should subscribe to a professional model of community care and, as far as possible, resist the tendency to adopt an administrative approach. A professional model is exploratory, holistic, integrative and therapeutic and is based on an understanding of the complex interconnected nature of needs for many older people. Table 9.2 describes the essential elements of a professional model of community care and illustrates the contrast with the administrative model. Within a professional approach, the scope and context of the assessment/care management processes are elaborative and the level of skill required from the practitioner will vary but will certainly involve on occasions a high level of ability to integrate a range of diverse skills within the user–practitioner relationship. The model is user-oriented in terms of process, content and evaluation: effectiveness is measured by user satisfaction and outcome.

The extent to which a professional model can be implemented in the context of the separation of purchaser and provider functions will depend upon the scope which exists for practitioners to influence *qualitatively* how the various elements of the assessment, care management and service delivery process are executed. While it may not be possible for the practitioner or manager to reconnect these elements within a particular organizational structure, the professional helper does have some power to determine how limited or extensive, how simple or complex, how reduced or elaborative his or her own particular function is defined and executed. By adopting a professional approach whenever possible, the practitioner can seek to minimize the trend towards, and impact of, an administrative model of community care.

2 *Assessment.* It is especially crucial that practitioners undertaking assessment work should adopt a holistic, elaborative approach and, where appropriate, the kind of comprehensive framework developed in Chapter 5. The point has already been made that assessment is the catalyst to the entire process and the way in which individual assessments are conducted, recorded and collated will have a major influence on the extent to which the community care process is either organizationally-oriented or user-oriented, resource-led or needs-led. A particular issue of relevance is that of unmet need. While most authorities are trying to gain a measure of the extent to which current services are adequate, practice remains varied in terms of the extent to which this is a measure of 'service deficit as opposed to unmet need and whether they record at the aggregate as well as the individual level' (Lewis 1994: 3).

However, as Chapter 1 has made clear, a picture of the aggregate level and types of unmet need must be the essential bedrock of the process of planning, commissioning and contracting upon which the structural edifice of community care is based. The aggregate picture can only be achieved if individual practitioners identify clearly unmet needs arising from comprehensive needs-based assessments. Thus, the *quality* of individual assessments is a crucial factor in determining the overall extent to which, over a period of time, a resource-rich local service context may develop. Improving the scope and quality of assessment practice is a necessary but not a sufficient condition for quality of service overall. However, it is clear that if assessments are limited or resource-led, the information upon which a call for improvement and development could be based will not exist.

3 *Address inequalities.* Biggs (1990) has highlighted the inherent tension between the stated objectives of community care and the likely outcomes in practice. In particular, he has questioned the extent to which the mechanisms for implementation are designed to locate user need within the wider context of social inequality and social problems. The individualization of need, which is at the heart of the care management processes, is not designed to integrate within those processes an understanding of the extent to which structural inequality and discriminatory attitudes have contributed to a particular set of circumstances. This emphasizes the points made above about the need for practitioners to adopt a comprehensive anti-discriminatory approach to their assessment work in particular.

However, the inherent tendency to individualize need is significant not only because it dislocates the elderly person from his or her social and historical contexts. It also means that the current arrangements for service provision are unlikely to include as an objective the reduction of inequality. Thus, the outcome of community care is expressed only in terms of meeting individual need, not in relation to the particular needs which may arise from a collective experience of old age through class, race or gender. The anti-discriminatory practitioner can begin to broaden the agenda by addressing issues of inequality within the assessment/care management process and by including consideration of such issues and their implications for particular older people and carers within their case recording and other written documents, as appropriate.

4 *Older people in minority ethnic groups.* In addition to the broad remit to address issues of inequality, particular focus must be given to older people in minority ethnic groups, not least because they are a sizeable minority whose needs remain largely unrecognized, certainly within the statutory sector (Anwal Bhalla and Blakemore 1981; Atkin and Rollings 1993). Black and Asian older people and carers are comparatively invisible as service users, a situation which has been tolerated and justified by the erroneous assumption that minority ethnic groups of people are characterized by close extended family networks within which elders are cared for (Barker 1984). Practitioners and managers must be aware of the under-representation of older people from minority ethnic groups and give particular attention to the importance of reaching out into these communities (1) to begin to understand the nature and level of need and (2) to develop appropriate services.

5 *User and carer participation.* The development of meaningful ways of enabling older people and carers to participate in, and be central to, the processes of assessment and care management is fundamental to good practice (Marsh and Fisher 1992). This imperative will not be met by the introduction of standardized procedures alone. For example, the routine sending of a completed assessment form to an older person may symbolize user rights but does not, *per se*, operationalize the concept of rights in a meaningful, valid way, particularly if the user has not been fully involved in the process or cannot interpret the implications of the written assessment when it arrives. The importance of user and carer participation, not only in the formulation of their own care packages, but also in the policy-making and planning processes, has to be incorporated into the attitudes of all professionals and integrated into the service delivery system if it is to be achieved (Twigg 1993).

6 *Quality.* Concern about quality must be at the heart of the anti-discriminatory approach to community care for older people. However, as this book has tried to demonstrate throughout, quality of outcome cannot be separated, either conceptually or in practice, from quality of process. In other words, the *way* things are done has a profound impact on the effectiveness and quality of the outcome. The end is partly determined by the means. To this extent, practitioners can have an important influence on the overall quality of an older person's experience of the service system by ensuring their own practice incorporates as far as possible the values and principles of an enabling, anti-discriminatory approach.

References

Allen, I. (ed.) (1990). *Care Managers and Case Management*. London: Policy Studies Institute.

Anwal Bhalla, A. and Blakemore, K. (1981). *Elders of the Ethnic Minority Groups*. Birmingham: All Faiths for One Race.

Arber, S. and Ginn, J. (1991). *Gender and Later Life*. London: Sage.

Association of Directors of Social Services (1991). *Adults at Risk – Guidance for Directors*. Stockport: ADSS.

Atchley, R. (1989). A continuity theory of normal aging. *The Gerontologist, 29*, 183–90.

Atkin, K. and Rollings, J. (1993). *Community Care in a Multi-Racial Britain*. London: HMSO.

Audit Commission (1986). *Making a Reality of Community Care*. London: HMSO.

Baker, A.A. (1975). Granny battering. *Modern Geriatrics, 5*(8), 20–4.

Barker, J. (1984). *Black and Asian Old People in Britain*. London: Age Concern England.

Beardshaw, V. (1990). Clearing the mystery. *Community Care*, 28 June.

Beardshaw, V. and Towell, D. (1990). *Assessment and Case Management*. Briefing Paper No. 11. London: King's Fund.

Beaver, M.L. (1991). Life review/reminiscent therapy. In P.K.H. Kim (ed.), *Serving the Elderly: Skills for Practice*, pp. 67–88. New York: Walter de Gruyter.

Bennett, G. and Kingston, P. (1993). *Elder Abuse: Concepts, Theories and Interventions*. London: Chapman and Hall.

Beresford, P. and Croft, S. (1994). A participatory approach to social work. In C. Hanvey and T. Philpot (eds), *Practising Social Work*. London: Routledge.

Biegel, D.E., Shore, B.K. and Gordon, E. (1984). *Building Support Networks for the Elderly*. London: Sage.

Biggs, S. (1990). Consumers, care management and inspection: Obscuring social deprivation and need. *Critical Social Policy, 10*(3), 23–38.

Biggs, S. (1993). *Understanding Ageing*. Milton Keynes: Open University Press.

Biggs, S. and Phillipson, C. (1992). *Understanding Elder Abuse*. Trowbridge: Longman.

Bigot, A. (1974). The relevance of American life satisfaction indices for research on British subjects before and after retirement. *Age and Ageing, 3*, 113–21.

Black, J. *et al.* (1983). *Social Work in Context*. London: Tavistock.

Blackburn, C. (1991). *Poverty and Health*. Buckingham: Open University Press.

Blakemore, K. (1985). Inequalities in old age: Some comparisons between Britain and the United States. *Journal of Applied Gerontology, 4*(1), 86–101.

Blakemore, K. and Boneham, M. (1994). *Age, Race and Ethnicity*. Buckingham: Open University Press.

Bond, J. and Coleman, P. (1990). *Ageing in Society*. London: Sage.

Bornat, J. (1994). *Reminiscence Reviewed: Perspectives, Evaluations, Achievements*. Buckingham: Open University Press.

Boulton, J., Gully, V., Matthews, L. and Gearing, B. (1989). *Developing the Biographical Approach in Practice with Older People*. Project Paper No. 7 of the Gloucester Care of Elderly People at Home Project. Milton Keynes: The Open University, School of Health, Welfare and Community Education.

Bowl, R. (1986). Social work and old people. In C. Phillipson and A. Walker (eds), *Ageing and Social Policy: A Critical Assessment*, pp. 128–45. Aldershot: Gower.

Breckman, R.S. and Adelman, R.D. (1988). *Strategies for Helping Victims of Elder Mistreatment*. London: Sage.

Briggs, R. (1990). Biological ageing. In J. Bond and P. Coleman (eds), *Ageing in Society*, pp. 53–67. London: Sage.

Bromley, D.R. (1988). *Human Ageing*, 3rd edn. London: Penguin.

Brown, A. (1986). *Groupwork*. London: Heinemann Educational.

Budge, M. (1989). *A Wealth of Experience: A Guide to Activities for Older People*. London: Jessica Kingsley.

Burack-Weiss, A. and Brennan, F.C. (1991). *Gerontological Social Work Supervision*. London: Haworth Press.

Burnside, I.M. (1978). *Working with the Elderly: Group Process and Techniques*. North Scituate, MA: Duxbury.

Bury, M. and Holme, A. (1991). *Life After Ninety*. London: Routledge.

Butler, R.N. (1963). The life review: An interpretation of reminiscence in the aged. *Psychiatry, 26*, 65–76.

Butler, R.N. (1974). Successful ageing and the role of life review. *Journal of the American Geriatrics Society, 22*(12), 529–35.

Bytheway, B. and Johnson, J. (1990). On defining ageism. *Critical Journal of Social Policy, 10*(2), 27–39.

Bytheway, B., Keil, T., Allatt, P. and Bryman, A. (1990). *Becoming and Being Old*. London: Sage.

Cambridge, P. (1992). Case management in community services: Organisational responses. *British Journal of Social Work, 22*, 495–517.

Challis, D. (1987). Case management and consumer choice: The Kent Community Care Scheme. In D. Clode, C. Parker and S. Etherington (eds), *Towards the Sensitive Bureaucracy: Consumers, Welfare and the New Pluralism*. Aldershot: Gower.

Challis, D. and Davies, B. (1986). *Case Management in Community Care*. Aldershot: Gower.

Challis, D., Darton, R., Johnson, L. and Traske, K. (1990). *The Darlington Community Care Project: Supporting Elderly People at Home*. Canterbury: Personal Social Services Research Unit, University of Kent.

Charlesworth, A., Wilkin, D. and Durie, A. (1984). *Carers and Services: A Comparison of Men and Women Caring for Dependent People*. Manchester: Equal Opportunities Commission.

Clarke, M. and Stewart, J.D. (1990). *General Management in Local Government: Getting the Balance Right*. Harlow: Longman.

Clayton, V.P. and Birren, J.E. (1980). The development of wisdom across the lifespan: A reexamination of an ancient topic. In P.B. Bates and O.G. Brim (eds), *Life-Span Development and Behaviour*, Vol. 3. New York: Academic Press.

Cloke, C. (1983). *Old Age Abuse in the Domestics Setting: A Review*. London: Age Concern England.

Coleman, P.G. (1986). *Ageing and Reminiscence Processes: Social and Clinical Implications*. Chichester: John Wiley.

Coleman, P.G. (1994). Reminiscence within the study of ageing: The social significance of story. In J. Bornat (ed.), *Reminiscence Reviewed: Perspectives, Evaluations, Achievements*, pp. 8–20. Buckingham: Open University Press.

Coulshed, V. (1988). *Social Work Practice: An Introduction*. London: Macmillan.

Croft, S. (1992). Empowerment in action. *Community Care Supplement*, 26 March, pp. ii–iii.

Crossman, R.H.S. (1962). Old people. *New Statesman*, 28 December, p. 930.

CSO (1991). *Social Trends 21*. London: HMSO.

Cumming, E. and Henry, W.E. (1961). *Growing Old: The Process of Disengagement*. New York: Basic Books.

Dant, T. and Gearing, B. (1990). Key workers for elderly people in the community: Case managers and care coordinators. *Journal of Social Policy, 19*, 331–60.

Decalmer, P. and Glendenning, F. (eds) (1993). *The Mistreatment of Elderly People*. London: Sage.

Department of the Environment (1988). *English House Condition Survey, 1986*. London: HMSO.

Department of Health (1989a). *Caring for People*. Cmd. 849. London: HMSO.

Department of Health (1989b). *Doing it Better Together: A Report of Developments in Four Locations to Establish Local Procedures for Multidisciplinary Assessment of the Needs of Elderly People*. London: Social Services Inspectorate.

Department of Health (1989c). *Homes for Living In*. London: HMSO.

Department of Health (1991a). *Caring for People: Implementation Documents. Draft Guidance: Assessment and Care Management*. London: HMSO.

Department of Health (1991b). *Working Together*. London: HMSO.

Department of Health (1991c). *Care Management and Assessment: Managers' Guide*. London: HMSO.

Department of Health (1991d). *Care Management and Assessment: Practitioners' Guide*. London: HMSO.

Department of Health and Social Security (1978). *A Happier Old Age: A Discussion Document*. London: HMSO.

Department of Health and Social Security (1986). Sir Roy Griffiths to review community care. *Press Release 86/410*. London: DHSS.

Donaldson, L. (1986). Health and social status of elderly Asians: A community survey. *British Medical Journal, 293*, 1079–81.

Eastman, M. (1984). *Old Age Abuse*. London: Age Concern England.

Egan, G. (1981). *The Skilled Helper: A Model for Systematic Therapy and Interpersonal Relating*. Monterey Park, CA: Brooks/Cole.

Erikson, E.H. (1965). *Childhood and Society*. Harmondsworth: Penguin.

Erikson, E.H. (1982). *The Life Cycle Completed: A Review*. New York: Norton.

Erikson, E.H., Erikson, J.M. and Kivnick, H.Q. (1986). *Vital Involvement in Old Age: The Experience of Old Age in Our Time*. New York: Norton.

Estes, C.L. (1979). *The Aging Experience*. San Francisco, CA: Jossey Bass.

Estes, C.L., Swan, J.H. and Gerard, L.E. (1984). Dominant and competing paradigms in gerontology: Towards a political economy of aging. In M. Minkler and C.L. Estes (eds), *Readings in the Political Economy of Aging*. Amityville, NY: Baywood Publishing.

Estes, C., Binney, E.A. and Culbertson, R.A. (1992). The gerontological imagination: Social influences on the development of gerontology, 1945–present. *International Journal of Aging and Human Development, 35*(1), 49–65.

Evandrou, M. and Falkingham, J. (1989). Benefit discrimination. *Community Care Supplement*, 25 May, pp. iii–iv.

Falkingham, J. (1989). Dependency and ageing in Britain: A re-examination of the evidence. *Journal of Social Policy, 18*(2), 211–33.

Falkingham, J. and Victor, C.R. (1991). The myth of the woopie?: Incomes, the elderly and targetting welfare. *Ageing and Society, 11*, 471–93.

Faragher, T. (1978). *Notes on the Evaluation of Residential Settings.* Publication No. 2, pp. 59–85. Birmingham: Clearing House for Local Authority Social Services Research.

Feil, N. (1982). *Validation: The Feil Method. How to Help Disorientated Old-Old.* Cleveland, OH: Edward Feil Publications.

Feil, N. (1991). Validation therapy. In P.K.H. Kim (ed.), *Serving the Elderly: Skills for Practice*, pp. 89–115. New York: Walter de Gruyter.

Felce, D. and Jenkins, J. (1978). *Engagement in Activities by Old People in Residential Care.* Health Care Evaluation Research Team, Report No. 50. Southampton: University of Southampton.

Finch, J. and Groves, D. (1985). Old girl, old boy: Gender divisions in social work with the elderly. In E. Brook and A. Davis (eds), *Women, the Family and Social Work*, pp. 92–111. London: Tavistock.

Fisher, M. (1990a). Care management and social work: Clients with dementia. *Practice, 4*(4), 229–41.

Fisher, M. (1990b). *Partnership Practice with Clients with Dementia.* Bradford: Social Work in Partnership, University of Bradford.

Fisher, M. (1990c). *Partnership Practice and Carers.* Bradford: Social Work in Partnership, University of Bradford.

Fisher, M. (1991). Defining the practice content of care managment. *Social Work and Social Sciences Review, 2*(3), 204–30.

Flynn, N. and Common, R. (1990). *Contracts for Community Care.* London: London Business School/HMSO.

Ford, J. and Sinclair, R. (1987). *Sixty Years On: Women Talk about Old Age.* London: The Women's Press.

Francis, J. (1993). Preventive assessment. *Community Care*, 29 July, p. 8.

Franklyn, A. (1992). A quality of life. *Community Care*, 24 September, pp. v–vi.

Fries, J.F. (1989). The compression of morbidity: Near or far. *Milbank Quarterly, 67*(2), 208–32.

Froggatt, A. (1988). Self-awareness in early dementia. In B. Gearing, M. Johnson and T. Heller (eds), *Mental Health Problems in Old Age*, pp. 131–6. Chichester: John Wiley.

Froggatt, A. (1990). *Family Work and Elderly People.* Basingstoke: Macmillan.

Garland, J. (1994). What splendour, it all coheres: Life review therapy with older people. In J. Bornat (ed.), *Reminiscence Reviewed: Perspectives, Evaluations, Achievements*, pp. 21–31. Buckingham: Open University Press.

Gearing, B. and Coleman, P. (in press). Biographical assessment in community care. In J. Birren, J.E. Ruth, J.J.F. Shroots and T. Svensson (eds), *Aging and Biography: Explorations in Adult Development.* New York: Springer.

Gearing, B. and Dant, T. (1990). Doing biographical research. In S. Peace (ed.), *Researching Social Gerontology*, pp. 143–59. London: Sage.

Gibson, F. (1994). What can reminiscence contribute to people with dementia? In J. Bornat (ed.), *Reminiscence Reviewed: Perspectives, Evaluations, Achievements*, pp. 46–60. Buckingham: Open University Press.

Glendenning, F. (1993). What is elder abuse and neglect. In P. Delcalmer and F. Glendenning (eds), *The Mistreatment of Elderly People*, pp. 1–34. London: Sage.

Greengross, S. (ed.) (1986). *The Law and Vulnerable Elderly People.* London: Age Concern England.

Griffiths, R. (1988). *Community Care: Agenda for Action.* London: HMSO.

Grundy, E. (1991). Age-related change in later life. In M. Murphy and J. Holscraft (eds), *Population Research in Britain.* London: Population Investigation Committee.

Gubrium, J.F. (1973). *The Myth of the Golden Years: A Socio-Environmental Theory of Aging*. Springfield, IL: Charles C. Thomas.

Hancock, B.L. (1987). *Social Work with Older People*. Englewood Cliffs, NJ: Prentice-Hall.

Harris, J. and Hopkins, T. (1994). Beyond ageism: Reminiscence groups and the development of anti-discriminatory social work education and practice. In J. Bornat (ed.), *Reminiscence Reviewed: Perspectives, Evaluations, Achievements*, pp. 74–88. Buckingham: Open University Press.

Hashimi, J. (1991). Counselling older adults. In P.K.H. Kim (ed.), *Serving the Elderly: Skills for Practice*, pp. 33–49. New York: Walter de Gruyter.

Haskey, J. (1989). Families and households of the ethnic minority and white populations of Great Britain. *Population Trends, 57*, 8–19.

Haskey, J. (1990). The ethnic minority population of Great Britain: Estimates by ethnic group and country of birth. *Population Trends, 60*, 35–8.

Havighurst, R.J. (1968). Personality and patterns of aging. *The Gerontologist, 8*, 20–3.

Hemmings, S. (1985). *A Wealth of Experience*. London: Pandora Press.

Hendricks, J. (1992). Generations and the generation of theory in social gerontology. *International Journal of Aging and Human Development, 35*(1), 31–47.

Hendricks, J. and Leedham, C.A. (1991). Theories of aging implications for human services. In P.K.H. Kim (ed.), *Serving the Elderly: Skills for Practice*, pp. 1–25. New York: Walter de Gruyter.

Henwood, M. and Wicks, M. (1985). Community care, family trends and social change. *Quarterly Journal of Social Affairs, 1*, 357–71.

Hickey, T. (1992). The continuity of gerontological themes. *International Journal of Aging and Human Development, 35*(1), 7–17.

Hocking, E.D. (1988). Miscare – a form of abuse in the elderly. *Update*, 15 May, pp. 2411–19.

Homer, A. and Gilleard, C. (1990). Abuse of elderly people and their carers. *British Medical Journal, 301*, 1359–62.

Howe, D. (1987). *An Introduction to Social Work Theory*. Aldershot: Wildwood House.

Hughes, B. (1990). Quality of life. In S. Peace (ed.), *Researching Social Gerontology*, pp. 46–58. London: Sage.

Hughes, B. (1993). A model for the comprehensive assessment of older people and their carers. *British Journal of Social Work, 23*, 345–64.

Hughes, B. and Mtezuka, E.M. (1992). Social work and older women. In M. Langan and L. Day (eds), *Women, Oppression and Social Work*, pp. 220–41. London: Routledge and Kegan Paul.

Hughes, B. and Wilkin, D. (1980). *Residential Care of the Elderly: A Review of the Literature*. Research Report No. 2. Manchester: Departments of Psychiatry and Community Medicine, University of Manchester.

Hull, R.H. and Griffin, K.M. (eds) (1989). *Communication Disorders in Aging*. London: Sage.

Hull, R.H. (1989). The hearing impaired older adult. In R.H. Hull and K.M. Griffin (eds), *Communication Disorders in Aging*, pp. 91–102. London: Sage.

Humphries, R. (1992). Champions of change. *Community Care*, 29 October, pp. 7–8.

Hunt, A. (1978). *The Elderly at Home*. London: HMSO.

Hunter, D.J. and Judge, K. (1988). Griffiths and Community Care: Meeting the Challenge. London: King's Fund Institute.

Huxley, P. (1993). Case management and care management in community care. *British Journal of Social Work, 23*, 365–81.

Johnson, M.L. (1976). That was your life: A biographical approach to later life. In J.M.A. Munnicks and W.J.A. van den Heuval (eds), *Dependency and Interdependency in Old Age*, pp. 147–61. The Hague: Martinus Nijhoff.

Johnson, P. and Falkingham, J. (1992). *Ageing and Economic Welfare*. London: Sage.

Jung, C.G. (1972). The transcendent function. In H. Read, M. Fordham, G. Adler and W. McGuire (eds), *The Structure of the Psyche, 2nd edn*. Volume 8 of the Collected Works of C.G. Jung. London: Routledge and Kegan Paul.

Key, M. (1989). The practice of assessing elders. In O. Stevenson (ed.), *Age and Vulnerability*, pp. 66–80. London: Edward Arnold.

Kim, P.K.H. (ed.) (1991). *Serving the Elderly: Skills for Practice*. New York: Walter de Gruyter.

Kitwood, T. and Bredin, K. (1992). Towards a theory of dementia care: Personhood and wellbeing. *Ageing and Society, 12*(3), 269–87.

Klein, W.H., Leshan, E.J. and Furman, S.S. (1965). *Promoting Mental Health of Older People Through Group Methods: A Practical Guide*. New York: Manhattan Society for Mental Health.

Knapp, M., Netten, A. and Beecham, J. (1993). Costing community care. In A. Netten and J. Beecham (eds), *Costing Community Care: Theory and Practice*, pp. 1–5. Aldershot: PSSRU/Ashgate Publishing.

Knight, B. (1986). *Psychotherapy with Older Adults*. London: Sage.

Lakatta, E.G. (1985). Heart and circulation. In C.E. Finch and E.L. Scheider (eds), *Handbook of the Biology of Aging*. New York: Van Nostrand Reinhold.

Lamb, H. (1981). Therapist case managers: More than brokers of service. *Hospital and Community Psychiatry, 31*, 759–64.

Langan, M. and Day, L. (1992). *Women, Oppression and Social Work*. London: Routledge.

Lart, R. and Means, R. (1992). Positive changes. *Community Care*, 17 December, p. 21.

Levin, E., Sinclair, I. and Gorbach, P. (1988). *Families, Services and Confusion in Old Age*. Aldershot: Gower.

Lewis, J. (1994). Care management and the social services: Reconciling the irreconcilable. *Generations Review, 4*(1), 2–4.

Liang, J., Dvorkin, L., Kahana, E. and Mazian, F. (1980). Social integration and morale: A re-examination. *Journal of Gerontology, 35*, 746–57.

Lishman, J. (1994). *Communication in Social Work*. London: Macmillan.

Longino, C.F. and Kart, C.S. (1982). Explicating activity theory: A formal replication. *Journal of Gerontology, 37*, 713–22.

Lunt, B., Felce, D., Jenkins, J. and Powell, L. (1977). *Organising Recreational Activity Sessions in a Home for the Elderly Mental Infirm: The Effect of Different Levels of Staff Input on Resident Participation*. Health Care Evaluation Research Team. Research Report No. 130. Southampton: University of Southampton.

Macdonald, B. and Rich, C. (1984). *Look Me in the Eye*. London: The Women's Press.

MacIntyre, S. (1977). Old age as a social problem. In R. Dingwall, C. Heath, M. Reid and M. Stacy (eds), *Health Care and Health Knowledge*, pp. 41–61. London: Croom Helm.

MacLennan, B.W., Saul, S and Weiner, M.D. (eds) (1988). *Group Psychotherapies for the Elderly*. Madison, WI: International Universities Press.

Malin, N. (ed.) (1994). *Implementing Community Care*. Buckingham: Open University Press.

Markides, K.S. (ed.) (1989). *Aging and Health: Perspectives on Gender, Race, Ethnicity and Class*. Newbury Park, CA: Sage.

Marsh, P. and Fisher, M. (1992). *Good Intentions: Developing Partnership in Social Services*. York: Community Care and Joseph Rowntree Foundation.

Marshall, M. (ed.) (1993). *Dementia*. London: Jessica Kingsley.

Matthews, S. H. (1979). *The Social World of Old Women*. Beverley Hills, CA: Sage.

Mayer, J.E. and Timms, N. (1969). *The Client Speaks*. London: Routledge and Kegan Paul.

McCreadie, C. (1991). *Elder Abuse: An Exploratory Study*. London: Age Concern England/ Institute of Gerontology.

Means, R. (1981). *Community Care and Meals on Wheels*. Working Paper No. 21. Bristol: University of Bristol, School for Advanced Urban Studies.

Merriman, S.B. (1989). The structure of simple reminiscence. *Gerontologist, 29*, 761–7.

Molinari, V. and Reichlin, R.E. (1985). Life review reminiscence in the elderly: A review of the initiative. *International Journal of Aging and Human Development, 20*, 81–92.

Moore, J. (Secretary of State for Social Services) (1989). *Transcript of Address to Help the Aged Sheltered Housing Conference*, 5 June 1989. London: Help the Aged.

Morris, J. (1992). Us and them? Feminist research, community care and disability. *Critical Social Policy, 33*, 22–39.

Morris, J. (1993). Involving service users. In The Next Key Tasks. *Community Care*, p. 1 (suppl.).

Moxley, D.P. (1989). *The Practice of Case Management*. London: Sage.

National Association of Race Equality Advisers (not dated). *Black Community Care Charter*. Birmingham: Race Relations Unit/NAREA.

National Association of Social Workers (ed.) (1963). *Social Group Work with Older People*. New York: NASW.

Neill, J. (1989). *Assessing Elderly People for Residential Care: A Practical Guide*. London: National Institute of Social Workers.

Nelson-Jones, R. (1983). *Practical Counselling Skills*. New York: Holt, Reinhart and Winston.

Neugarten, D.L., Havighurst, R.J. and Mobin, S.S. (1961). The measurement of life satisfaction. *Journal of Gerontology, 16*, 134–43.

Norman, A. (1979). *Rights and Risk: A Discussion Document on Civil Liberty in Old Age*. London: Centre for Policy on Ageing.

Norman, A. (1985). *Triple Jeopardy: Growing Old in a Second Homeland*. London: Centre for Policy on Ageing.

Norman, A. (1987). *Aspects of Ageing: A Discussion Paper*. London: Centre for Policy on Ageing.

Norris, A. (1986). *Reminiscences with Elderly People*. London: Winslow Press.

Ogg, J. and Bennett, G.C.J. (1992) Elder abuse in Britain. *British Medical Journal, 24* October, pp. 998–9.

Ogg, J. and Munn-Giddings, C. (1993). Researching elder abuse. *Ageing and Society, 13*, 389–413.

O'Malley, H., Segars, H. and Perez, R. (1979). *Elder Abuse in Massachusetts: A Survey of Professionals and Paraprofessionals*. Boston, MA: Legal Research and Services for the Elderly.

Orme, J. and Glastonbury, B. (1993). *Care Management*. London: Macmillan.

OPCS (1982). *General Household Survey 1980*. London: HMSO.

OPCS (1989). *General Household Survey 1986*. London: HMSO.

OPCS (1990). *General Household Survey 1988*. London: OPCS.

OPCS (1991). *National Population Projections 1989 Based*. Series PP2 No. 17. London: HMSO.

Open University (1982). *Caring for Older People*. Course P650. Buckingham: The Open University.

Øvretreit, J. (1993). *Coordinating Community Care*. Buckingham: Open University Press.

Payne, M. (1986). *Social Care in the Community*. London: Macmillan.

Peace, S. (1986). The forgotten female: Social policy and older women. In C. Phillipson and A. Walker (eds), *Ageing and Social Policy: A Critical Assessment*, pp. 61–86. Aldershot: Gower.

Penhale, B. (1993). The abuse of elderly people: Considerations for practice. *British Journal of Social Work, 23*, 95–112.

Phillips, L. (1986). Theoretical explanations of elder abuse. In K. Pillemer and R. Wolfe (eds), *Elder Abuse: Conflict in the Family*. Dover, MA: Auburn House.

Phillipson, C. (1972). *Capitalism and the Construction of Old Age.* London: Macmillan.

Pillemer, K. (1986). Risk factors in elder abuse: Results from a case-control study. In K. Pillemer and R.S. Wolf (eds), *Elder Abuse: Conflict in the Family.* Dover, MA: Auburn House.

Pillemer, K.A. and Finkelhor, D. (1988). The prevalence of elder abuse in a random sample survey. *The Gerontologist, 28*(1), 51–7.

Pritchard, J. (1992). *The Abuse of Elderly People: A Handbook for Professionals.* London: Jessica Kingsley.

Rabbitt, P.M.A. (1988). Social psychology, neuroscience and cognitive psychology need each other (and gerontology needs all three of them). *The Psychologist: Bulletin of the British Psychological Society, 12,* 500–6.

Renshaw, J. (1988). Care in the community: Individual care planning and case management. *British Journal of Social Work, 18,* 79–105 (suppl.).

Renshaw, J., Hampson, R., Thomason, C., Darton, R., Judge, K. and Knapp, M. (1988). *Care in the Community: The First Steps.* Aldershot: Gower.

Riley, P. (1989). Professional dilemmas in elder abuse. Paper presented at a seminar on *Elder Abuse,* Welsh Association of Health Authorities, 28 September.

Rochdale Social Services Department (1993). *Working Together: Guidelines for Staff to Follow when Abuse of Older People is Suspected or Confirmed.* Rochdale: Rochdale Social Services Department.

Rogers, C. (1951a). *Client Centred Therapy.* London: Constable.

Rogers, C. (1951b). *On Becoming a Person.* London: Constable.

Rose, A.M. (1965). The subculture of aging: A framework in social gerontology. In A.M. Rose and W.A. Peterson (eds), *Older People and their Social World,* pp. 3–16. Philadelphia, PA: F.A. Davies.

Rose, S.R. (1991). Small group processes and interventions with the elderly. In P.K.H. Kim (ed.), *Serving the Elderly: Skills for Practice,* pp. 167–86. New York: Walter de Gruyter.

Rowlings, C. (1985). Practice in field care. In J. Lishman (ed.), *Research Highlights in Social Work 3: Developing Services for the Elderly,* 2nd edn. London: Kogan Page.

Sainsbury, E., Nixon, S. and Phillips, S. (1982). *Social Work in Focus: Clients' and Social Workers' Perspectives in Long Term Social Work.* London: Routledge.

Scrutton, S. (1989). *Counselling Older People.* London: Edward Arnold.

Silverstone, B. and Burack-Weiss, A. (1983). *Social Work Practice with the Frail Elderly and Their Families.* Springfield, IL: Charles C. Thomas.

Sinclair, I. and Gibb, I. (1990). *Interim Report on the Checklist Project.* York: University of York, Department of Social Policy and Social Work.

Social Services Inspectorate, Department of Health (1992). *Confronting Elder Abuse.* London: HMSO.

Social Services Inspectorate, Department of Health (1993). No longer afraid: The safeguard of older people in domestic settings. *National Practice Guidelines.* London: HMSO.

Stevenson, O. (1989). *Age and Vulnerability.* London: Edward Arnold.

Stokes, G. (1992). *On Being Old: The Psychology of Later Life.* London: Falmer Press.

Strehler, B.L. (1962). *Time, Cells and Aging.* New York: Academic Press.

Stuart-Hamilton, I. (1994). *The Psychology of Ageing,* 2nd edn. London: Jessica Kingsley.

Thienhaus, O.L., Conter, E.A. and Bosmann, H.B. (1986). Sexuality and ageing. *Ageing and Society, 6,* 39–54.

Thompson, N. (1993). *Anti-Discriminatory Practice.* London: Macmillan.

Thompson, P. (1992). 'I don't feel old': Subjective ageing and the search for meaning in later life. *Ageing and Society, 12,* 23–47.

Tinker, A. (1992). *Elderly People in Modern Society,* 3rd edn. London: Longman.

Titmuss, R.M. (1955). Pensions, systems and population change. *Political Quarterly, 26,* 152–66.

Tobin, S.S. (1991). *Personhood in Advance Old Age*. New York: Springer.

Townsend, P. (1981). The structured dependency of the elderly: A creation of social policy in the twentieth century. *Ageing and Society, 1*(1), 5–28.

Townsend, P. and Davidson, N. (1982). *Inequalities of Health*. London: Penguin.

Twigg, J. (1993). Integrating carers into the service system: Six strategic responses. *Ageing and Society, 13*, 141–70.

Victor, C.R. (1991). *Health and Health Care in Later Life*. Milton Keynes: Open University Press.

Victor, C.R. (1994). *Old Age in Modern Society: A Textbook of Social Gerontology*, 2nd edn. London: Croom Helm.

Walker, A. (1980). The social creation of poverty and dependency in old age. *Journal of Social Policy, 9*, 49–75.

Walker, A. (1981). Towards a political economy of old age. *Ageing and Society, 1*, 73–94.

Walker, A. (1987). The poor relation: Poverty among old women. In C. Glendinning and J. Millar (eds), *Women and Poverty in Britain*, pp. 178–98. Brighton: Wheatsheaf.

Walker, A. (1988). The financial resources of the elderly. In S. Baldwin, G. Parker and R. Walker (eds), *Social Security and Community Care*, pp. 45–73. Aldershot: Avebury.

Walker, A. (1990). Poverty and inequality in old age. In J. Bond and P. Coleman (eds), *Ageing in Society*, pp. 280–303. London: Sage.

Warnes, A. and Law, C.M. (1984). The elderly population of Britain. *Transactions of the Institute of British Geographers, New Series, 9* (1), 37–59.

Wilkin, D. and Hughes, B. (1986). The elderly and the health service. In C. Phillipson and A. Walker (eds), *Ageing and Society: A Critical Assessment*, pp. 163–83. Aldershot: Gower.

Wilkin, D. and Hughes, B. (1987). Residential care of elderly people: The consumers' views. *Ageing and Society, 7*, 175–201.

Wilson, G. (1993). Users and providers: Different perspectives on community care services. *Journal of Social Policy, 22*(4), 507–26.

Wistow, G., Knapp, M., Hardy, B. and Allen, C. (1994). *Social Care in a Mixed Economy*. Buckingham: Open University Press.

Working Party on Joint Planning (1985). *Progress in Partnership*. London: Department of Health and Social Security (Community Services Division).

Index